Praise for

5-HTP

and Michael Murray, N.D.

"A clear and practical guide for naturally and safely increasing serotonin levels and treating a wide variety of symptoms ranging from excess body fat to PMS . . . I recommend it highly."
—Christiane Northrup, M.D., author of *Women's Bodies, Women's Wisdom*

"Books by Dr. Michael Murray are always precise, well documented and enormously helpful. *5-HTP: The Natural Way to Overcome Depression, Obesity, and Insomnia* is no exception. Those who read and act on the information in this book will benefit well beyond their expectations."
—Julian Whitaker, M.D., author of *Dr. Whitaker's Guide to Natural Healing*

"Michael Murray's book is absolutely outstanding. I would highly recommend this book to any complimentary health care provider interested in alternatives for improving quality of life in people afflicted with depression, anxiety, and insomnia."
—Stephen T. Sinatra, M.D., author of *Optimum Health*

"5-HTP prevents and controls depression, insomnia, and aggression, as well as appetite and weight, particularly for 'carbohydrate cravers' . . . Infinitely better than a 'wonder drug,' 5-HTP is a 'miracle molecule,' an integral part of the miracle of life on Earth."
—Jonathan V. Wright, M.D., medical director, Tahoma Clinic, Kent, Washington

"Reading 5-HTP is like a leisurely consultation with an enormously skilled and caring doctor. You will gain a rare understanding of depression, as well as obesity and insom-

nia, and learn exactly how to help yourself . . . A must for your library and anyone you care about."
—Jane Heimlich, author of *What Your Doctor Won't Tell You*

"Dr. Murray has written an exceptional book on 5-HTP that will be of invaluable benefit to consumers and practitioners alike."
—Alexander G. Schauss, Ph.D., American Institute for Biosocial Research, Inc.

"We're all searching for a supplement that is safe, readily available, and most of all, that can help us feel better. Look no more: Dr. Michael Murray has found it, and it is 5-HTP."
—Jan McBarron, M.D., bariatric (weight loss) specialist

"Dr. Murray has presented convincing evidence that 5-HTP is an important alternative to potentially dangerous prescription drugs. Because 5-HTP can influence brain and body chemistry, I recommend that it be used under medical supervision."
—Alan R. Gaby, M.D., past president, American Holistic Medical Association

5-HTP

*The Natural Way
to Overcome
Depression, Obesity,
and Insomnia*

Michael T. Murray, N.D.

BANTAM BOOKS

NEW YORK   TORONTO   LONDON   SYDNEY   AUCKLAND

This edition contains the complete text
of the original hardcover edition.
NOT ONE WORD HAS BEEN OMITTED.

5-HTP
A Bantam Book

PUBLISHING HISTORY
Bantam hardcover edition published 1998
Bantam trade paperback edition / June 1999

*Grateful acknowledgment is made to the following for permission to reprint previously
published material:*

The National Mental Health Association for kindly supplying the Depression Questionnaire in Chapter Two.

The Metropolitan Life Insurance Company, Statistical Bulletin, which provided the Metropolitan Life Insurance Company Height and Weight Table used in Chapter Three.

Book design by Karin Batten
Library of Congress Catalog Card Number: 97-46868

ISBN 0-553-37946-1

Published simultaneously in the United States and Canada

Bantam Books are published by Bantam Books, a division of Random House, Inc. Its
trademark, consisting of the words "Bantam Books" and the portrayal of a rooster, is
Registered in U.S. Patent and Trademark Office and in other countries. Marca Registrada.
Bantam Books, 1540 Broadway, New York, New York 10036.

PRINTED IN THE UNITED STATES OF AMERICA

10 9 8 7 6 5 4 3 2 1

To my son, Zachary Michael Murray

CONTENTS

ACKNOWLEDGMENTS

The first person I absolutely must acknowledge is my beautiful wife, Gina. The gestation of this book coincided with her pregnancy with our second child, our son Zachary. Gina endured little help from me during the first few weeks of Zach's life as I worked diligently to write this book in a timely fashion. Gina, I appreciate and love you intensely. I also must give thanks to my wonderful little three-year-old, Alexa. Thank you, Lexi, for brightening my world and providing valuable nourishment to my soul with our play time.

Next, I would like to acknowledge my agent, Bonnie Solow, of New Media Marketing. Her assistance, support, and friendship were very much appreciated during the course of this book. Thank you, Bonnie.

I also want to thank my editors at Bantam, Toni Burbank and Emily Heckman, for helping me to mold this book into its final version and for introducing me to Ron Schaumburg, to whom I am also extremely indebted, for his enormous contribution in helping translate my original draft into a much more "reader friendly" form. Thank you Toni, Emily, and Ron.

And finally, I would like to thank all those dedicated scientists who have studied 5-HTP and L-tryptophan over the years. Their discoveries have definitely enriched the lives of many.

5-HTP

INTRODUCTION

Chances are that you, like millions of other Americans, are suffering from health problems that are a direct consequence of our stressed-out, modern way of living. Many people today awaken in the morning feeling unrested after a night of fitful sleep. They drag themselves through the day feeling moody, tired, achy. Succumbing to their cravings for sugary, carbohydrate-laden foods, they put on pounds that only add to their body's burden. They shuttle from doctor to doctor seeking pills that will lift them from their depression, help them control their weight, put a stop to their pounding headaches and the nagging aches in their muscles and joints, and finally get a good night's sleep.

It may surprise you to learn that all of these serious, debilitating complaints can arise from a problem with a single, powerful chemical the body needs to function normally. That chemical is serotonin.

Serotonin is absolutely essential for your brain—and thus your body—to function properly. Serotonin is a neurotransmitter, a chemical that carries vital signals from one cell to the next. Without adequate levels of serotonin, those signals cannot move at the proper speed or intensity. What's more, serotonin acts as a kind of master control chemical. The activities of many other important brain compounds—including those that govern your muscle movements, your state of alertness, your mental activity, even your ability to fall asleep—depend on serotonin.

But poor diet, lack of exercise, use of harmful substances such as caffeine or alcohol, and overall physical and emotional stress can rob your brain of the ability to make enough serotonin to meet your body's demands. This produces a range of significant complications: depression, obesity, insomnia, migraine headache, chronic fatigue. Increasingly, scientists, doctors, and other health experts around the world are coming to recognize that this group of complaints all arise from problems with basic brain chemistry. The disorder has a name: *serotonin deficiency syndrome*.

And here's the exciting news. All of these maladies can be corrected through the same technique: by raising serotonin levels.

Serotonin was first discovered about fifty years ago. Since then an enormous amount of research has been done to unlock the secrets of this multitalented molecule. In the past few decades, findings in the laboratory have led to the development of many potent serotonin-active compounds. Among these are Prozac, the popular antidepressant, which enhances the mood-regulating activity of serotonin; Imitrex, a treatment for migraine headaches, which works by activating serotonin nerve pathways to constrict blood vessels; and Redux, the appetite suppressant that was recently removed from the market, which controls eating by delivering a dose of serotonin to the appetite control centers in the brain. Other serotonin-altering drugs relieve anxiety, enhance sleep, and ease muscular and skeletal pain.

But these medical miracles come with a pretty high price tag. The side effects of synthetic serotonin drugs can be severe. To take just one example: In September 1997 Redux and its chemical cousin fenfluramine, part of the "fen-phen" combination, were yanked off the market. The reason? Doctors suddenly discovered these drugs had caused permanent damage to heart valves in as many as one third of the people who took them.

Fortunately, there's a better way to overcome serotonin deficiency. But because of the way the body makes neurotransmitters, you can't simply take a dose of serotonin as a pill or a tonic. What you can do, though, is provide your body with the raw material it needs to produce its own serotonin.

That raw material is called 5-hydroxytryptophan—5-HTP for short.

5-HTP is not a synthetic drug. It is a compound produced by the body from tryptophan, an amino acid found in many foods. It can be very difficult to consume enough tryptophan in the diet to overcome serotonin deficiency. However, 5-HTP can also be extracted from plants. This form of 5-HTP is now widely available— without a prescription—as a nutritional supplement. As you will learn in this book, 5-HTP promises to revolutionize the treatment of serotonin-related emotional and physical conditions.

In Europe, 5-HTP has been used for decades as an approved treatment for depression, sleep problems, weight loss, and other medical complaints. It is just now starting to sweep America. In my practice as a licensed physician, I have prescribed 5-HTP as part of overall therapy programs for hundreds of patients in just the past few years. The results I have seen have been tremendous: improved mood, better physical vitality, higher energy levels, a rediscovery of the basic joy of being alive.

Research into 5-HTP and serotonin is exploding. Throughout this book you will learn about the results of scientific and clinical studies, here and abroad, that are helping to unlock the secrets of 5-HTP. While there are many questions yet to explore, the evidence is clear: 5-HTP is a safe, natural way to boost brain serotonin levels. Use of 5-HTP has been shown to produce results equal to or better than those of standard synthetic drugs used in the treatment of problems arising from serotonin deficiency syndrome.

My goal in writing this book is to provide you with the information and guidance you need to understand what 5-HTP can do for you. Along the way I will explain some of the fascinating activity that takes place inside your brain and your body every second of every day. Understanding that process will help underscore your awareness of what a magnificent creation your body is, and how a deficiency in a single chemical substance—serotonin—can wreak such widespread havoc.

Just as important, you'll also discover how the safe and appropriate use of 5-HTP can produce dramatic results in the form of better mood, better sleep, less pain, and greater satisfaction with life.

CHAPTER 1

5-HTP AND THE SEROTONIN SYSTEM: AN OVERVIEW

The numbers are frightening:

- Each year, depression strikes ten million people in the United States. In the course of their lifetimes, one woman in every four and one man out of ten will develop depression.
- One out of three Americans weighs more than he or she should; many suffer from obesity that drastically increases their risk of heart disease, diabetes, or other life-threatening illnesses.
- Each year, one third of the people in this country experience prolonged periods of sleep disturbance serious enough to disrupt their mental or physical well-being or affect their performance during the day.
- One out of ten people (three times as many women as men) suffers from the searing pain of migraine headaches.

- Over five million Americans—again, most of them women—drag themselves through their days feeling an overwhelming sense of bone-wearying pain and muscle ache that overwhelms their whole body.

If misery loves company, then these people can take comfort in the fact that they are not alone in their unhappiness. They also have something else in common: Something is terribly wrong with their brain chemistry. Specifically, in many cases, all of the above conditions can arise from a single cause: abnormally low levels of a powerful and vital chemical called serotonin.

If you count yourself among any of the groups I've just described, I have some great news for you. In scientific laboratories all over the world, a growing body of exciting research is showing that it is possible to boost your serotonin levels safely, effectively—*without* dangerous drugs and *without* the risk of serious side effects.

Before I explain how, let's first take a look at how we human beings got ourselves into this sorry state of affairs. Then I'll take you on a fascinating journey inside the body so that you can see how the chemicals your brain needs are made and how they work. By the end of this chapter, you'll realize that serotonin deficiency syndrome is indeed a modern malady, a significant threat to health and well-being. It is a problem that calls for a modern— and natural—solution.

Stress and Your Brain

In many ways, the imbalance of brain chemistry is a tragic but predictable by-product of our contemporary, fast-paced, stressed-out way of living. Take diet, for example. You've heard the old expression "You are what you eat." Well, today many people in the United States and other Westernized countries eat diets that are not just unhealthy but downright deadly. We wolf down fast-food burgers, french fries, and fried chicken, all dripping with saturated fat and loaded with sodium. We turn up our nose at fresh fruits and vegetables so we can "save room for dessert." Because we crave sweets and other carbohydrates, we fill in the empty spaces in our tummy with candy bars and chips and other snacks. Instead of eating a balanced diet of nutritious foods, we grab processed, prepackaged, preservative-loaded items from the grocery store shelves and spend a fortune on vitamins and supplements to provide us with the nutrients we need.

It's not just the foods we eat (or don't eat) that contribute to the problem. It's our whole *pattern* of eating. Many of us skip breakfast and often lunch too, then gorge on huge dinners. Or we consume more calories than we need, and then we don't exercise enough to burn off the excess pounds that accumulate. Recent surveys report the alarming news that one out of three Americans, including children and teenagers, is overweight. We may diet for a while, but eventually our willpower crumbles and we revert to our old habits. The combination of poor nutrition, lousy eating habits, and yo-yo dieting adds up to one troublesome fact: We simply don't supply our bodies with the raw material we need to produce crucial brain chemicals, including serotonin.

Stress is another big factor. Many of us find it very hard to keep up with the daily grind. To make ends meet we work long hours, hold down two jobs, work nights and weekends. Nor have technological advances produced the savings in time we had been led to expect. Faxes, FedEx, E-mail, and "just-in-time" management and production only seem to increase the amount of work we're supposed to produce in the course of a day. Today, the concepts of the eight-hour day and the four-day work week seem as quaint and antiquated as the bustle and the top hat. As the Red Queen said to Alice in *Through the Looking-Glass,* "It takes all the running you can do, to keep in the same place."

But stress comes in many forms. Broadly speaking, a stressor is any factor that forces the body to respond and work harder just to maintain its equilibrium. Examples of stressors include prolonged exposure to heat and cold, coping with environmental toxins such as polluted air or chemical-laden water, and chronic physical ailments. Disturbances in our emotional well-being can also be a form of stress. Our moods and emotions are regulated by brain chemicals. Feeling constantly sad or depressed or angry takes a serious toll on the body, which tries constantly to adjust its chemical balance to counteract the damage.

To understand the impact of stress, try to recall the last time you experienced a moment of sudden, severe fright. Perhaps an oncoming car unexpectedly swerved into your lane, or you were startled by a loud noise coming from your child's bedroom. As you are no doubt aware, immediately after such a fright you feel a rush of energy. Your heart begins pounding, your palms sweat, your mind races—all systems go into a state of high alert. This is what biologists call the fight-or-flight response, and it results from a sudden surge of the hormone adrenaline. The role of adrenaline is to provide your body with the rush of energy it needs to cope with a sudden threat. Do you need to run away from the source of danger? Adrenaline gets your heart racing, your lungs pumping, and the muscles in your legs moving. Do you need to stand and fight? Adrenaline focuses your attention on the enemy, shortens your reaction time, and diverts body strength to the muscles you need for battle. When the danger passes, the brain adjusts the chemical balance to ratchet down the activity, calm your pounding heart, and restore your overall sense of equilibrium.

Clearly, adrenaline is a big asset when it comes to our dealing with immediate threats to our survival. But you wouldn't want to live constantly in such a state of all-out, all-systems-go arousal. It would be too exhausting. In a sense, however, that's exactly what happens when we endure chronic stress arising from the problems of daily living. Even mild stress activates the fight-or-flight response on some level. The longer we are forced to cope with stress, the more out of balance our brain chemistry becomes.

Another factor comes into play: our psychological skill at managing stress. Experts refer to this ability as our "coping style." Some people are able to handle a crisis with calm and poise.

Others confronted with the same problem throw up their hands and say, "I just can't deal with it." People who fail to develop a successful method of dealing with stress are more likely to turn to unhealthy strategies. Among the more common negative or destructive coping patterns are:

- Overeating
- Too much television
- Emotional outbursts
- Feelings of helplessness
- Overspending
- Chemical dependency (on legal or illegal drugs, alcohol, or tobacco)

→Cigarette smoking, alcohol abuse, a high sugar intake, blood sugar disturbances (hypoglycemia and diabetes), and excessive protein consumption all put tremendous stress on your body. Over time, this stress seriously impairs your ability to manufacture, and make use of, the necessary brain chemicals. By the same token, maintaining a healthy lifestyle, eating a nutritious and balanced diet, exercising, and learning effective stress management techniques can go a long way toward restoring optimal levels of neurotransmitters in the brain.

Making these adjustments in your life takes time and effort, but the results are well worth it. Meanwhile, there are steps you can take to help restore your body and your mind to a higher level of functioning. Before I explain how, let me take you on a quick tour of perhaps the most amazing landscape in the known universe: your brain.

Inside the Brain

All brain activity—every thought you have, every feeling and emotion, every order the brain sends to the organs and cells and fibers in your body—is the product of electrochemical signals. These signals zip along the brain's intricate and delicate network of specialized cells called neurons (Figure 1.1). The brain contains billions of these long, thin nerve cells.

Neurons have several parts. The *nucleus* is the "headquarters" of the cell, responsible for organizing and carrying out the cell's function. Stretching out from the nucleus is a long tail-like fiber called the *axon*. Electrical signals travel along the axon at nearly the speed of light, just as they do along the wires in your electrical appliances.

At the opposite end of the cell from the axon are branching fibers called *dendrites*. Seen under a microscope, dendrites look like the roots of a tree. Dendrites reach toward—but do not actually contact—the axons of one or more neighboring neurons. The microscopically small space between the dendrite and the axon is called the synaptic cleft or, more simply, the *synapse*.

Inside the dendrite are tiny pouches or sacs known as *vesicles*. Vesicles store the neuron's supply of special chemicals called *neurotransmitters,* which play a vital role in transmitting messages between the neurons of the brain.

The end of the axon, called the *axon terminal,* is wrapped in a thin membrane. When an electrical signal travels along the axon and reaches the terminal, it signals the vesicle to release some or all of its supply of neurotransmitter. Molecules of the chemical then flow through an opening in the membrane and float into the synapse.

The neurotransmitter "swims" in the fluid that flows through the synapse. Within a tiny fraction of a second, the molecules of neurotransmitter come into contact with a neighboring neuron (Figure 1.2). The surface of these neurons is studded with various protein molecules, which are called *receptors*.

There are many kinds of receptors. Like pieces of a jigsaw puzzle, each type of receptor has a unique shape that allows only certain types of molecules to attach to (or bind with) it. Thus a molecule of serotonin, for example, will bind only with a serotonin receptor. Once binding occurs, the neurotransmitter completes a

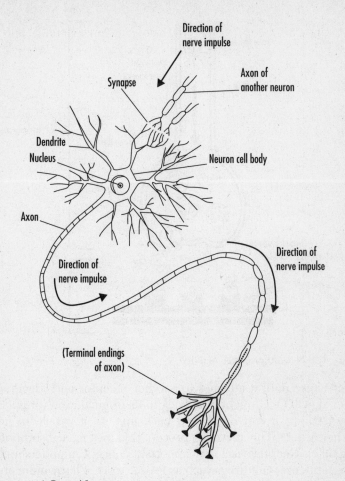

Figure 1.1: A Brain Neuron

circuit and stimulates an electrical current. The signal then flows along the axon of the neuron, triggering the release of still more neurotransmitters from other vesicles.

Once the neurotransmitter molecule has delivered its "message," it detaches from the receptor. A number of things can then happen. The neurotransmitter molecule can keep floating around

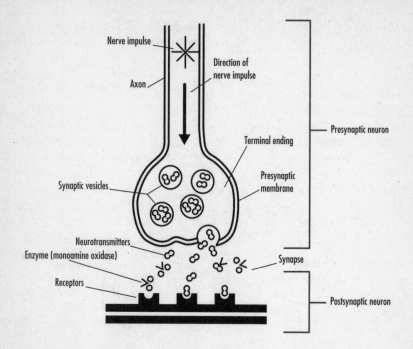

Figure 1.2: Neurotransmitter Activity

the synapse until it attaches to another receptor and triggers another signal. Or it might float back to its original axon (or another axon), where it can be sucked back up into a vesicle to await further orders. This recycling process is known as reabsorption or reuptake. (Reuptake is a very important concept in understanding how antidepressant drugs such as Prozac work. I'll say more about this in the next chapter.) Often the neurotransmitter comes into contact with another type of protein molecule known as an *enzyme*. Enzymes are like chemical scissors. Their job is to cut large molecules into smaller pieces. This, in turn, makes it easier for the body to metabolize (break down) and eliminate substances so it can maintain the chemical balance needed to function properly.

One other point is worth making. The term *neurotransmitter* generally refers to chemicals that produce their effects on cells that are neighboring or are very close by, such as the neurons. In contrast, a *hormone* is a chemical that is produced by one organ and then travels to tissues or organs elsewhere in the body to exert its effects. Many body chemicals, including serotonin and epinephrine, act both as neurotransmitters and as hormones.

To summarize: Nerve cells in the brain store neurotransmitters and release them in response to electrical signals. The neurotransmitters attach to receptors on neighboring cells. When they attach, they trigger another electrical signal, and the message continues to travel through the brain. Once the neurotransmitter has done its job, it either remains in circulation, gets sucked back up into a neuron, or is dissolved by an enzyme and flushed out of the body.

How Neurotransmitters Work

As you might imagine, given the complexity of this marvelous system, there are a number of factors that can affect the activity of neurotransmitters in the brain. For example, the amount of neurotransmitter molecules stored in the vesicles may be too high or too low. If your supply is depleted, then signals from the axon will not cause the release of neurotransmitter from the vesicle, just as plugging in a lamp won't give you light if the bulb is burned out. This particular problem—inadequate supply of neurotransmitters, especially serotonin—is the main focus of our discussion in this book.

Sometimes the neurons are overactive. By that I mean that they are *too* sensitive to electrical signals. The slightest nudge causes them to release more neurotransmitter than is needed to do the job. Too much serotonin operating in the synapse can cause feelings of sleepiness, loss of appetite, or other symptoms.

Another potential problem is that the "pump" that reabsorbs the neurotransmitter during reuptake may be defective. If too few neurotransmitter molecules are reabsorbed by the neuron, there won't be enough of the neurotransmitter available for release in response to the next signal from the axon.

Sometimes people have enzyme levels that are too high. This can occur as the result of a genetic problem or a chronic disease, such as a liver disorder. If too many enzymes are present, they may attack and destroy the neurotransmitter before it can reach the receptor to complete the circuit. As a result, not enough neurotransmitter reaches the receptor to keep the signal moving. Or the enzyme may cut apart so many neurotransmitter molecules that there are none left for reuptake. The net result is the same: abnormally low neurotransmitter levels and a severe imbalance of brain chemistry.

Another problem arises when other kinds of molecules block the receptor. If this happens, the neurotransmitter is prevented from binding effectively to the receptor and triggering its signal. Or it may be the case that the neuron is defective, unable to produce the right number or type of receptors. In such cases, the supply of neurotransmitter available in the brain might be adequate, but the molecules cannot find "parking spaces" and so they cannot deliver their messages. Some forms of brain damage can also disrupt the transmission process by weakening the electrical signals that travel along the axon or by severing the nerve fiber.

As you no doubt realize, there are a number of things that can go wrong with your brain's neurotransmitter system: bad wiring, faulty sockets, power shortages, short circuits. When neurotransmitters are not released in the right quantities, or if they can't reach their target and do their job, problems—many of them quite serious—can develop.

A Closer Look

Let's look a little more closely at these amazing and powerful chemicals, the neurotransmitters. These molecules play a number of very important roles in the brain. They regulate our moods, control various functions including appetite and sleep, and govern our response to pain.

Scientists have identified at least forty chemicals (some experts say there are hundreds) that work as messengers in the brain, and more are being discovered all the time. There are about ten major neurotransmitters, and they fall into three main groups: single amino acids, neuropeptides, and monoamines.

Of the three groups of neurotransmitters, amino acids are present in the brain in the highest amounts. To a chemist, an amino acid is a molecule that combines an amine group (one atom of nitrogen plus one or two atoms of hydrogen) and an acid group (one atom each of hydrogen and carbon plus two atoms of oxygen). Each amino acid also contains various other atoms arranged in specific and unique patterns. Amino acids act directly and rapidly on neurons. I'll say more about amino acids and their importance in the body shortly.

The second group of neurotransmitters are the neuropeptides. These proteins are chains made up of two or more amino acids. Although neuropeptides are found in lower concentrations in the brain than are the other two neurotransmitter groups, they are also the most powerful. [Examples of neuropeptides are endorphins and their cousins, the enkephalins. As I'll explain later, the main role of these neuropeptides is in managing the body's response to pain.]

The third group, and the ones of most interest to us in this book, are the monoamines. To a biochemist, the name indicates that these molecules include a single amine group. In addition, each monoamine contains various other molecules that give it unique properties. There are two main families of monoamine neurotransmitters: the catecholamines, which include dopamine, norepinephrine, and epinephrine (also called adrenaline); and the indoleamines, which include melatonin and the star of our show, serotonin.

Serotonin: The Brain's Master Molecule

Serotonin—which scientists also call 5-hydroxytryptamine, or 5-HT for short—plays many vital roles in brain chemistry.[1] Not only is it important in itself for controlling your moods and behavior, it also acts as a kind of chemical traffic cop that regulates the activity of many other neurotransmitters. If your serotonin levels are too low, then your brain and your entire body may perform poorly, just as the performance of the entire play suffers when the leading actor fails to make his entrance or remember his lines.

Scientists first discovered and isolated serotonin from the blood in the 1940s. Research since then confirms that serotonin has many important effects throughout the body. For example, serotonin is found in platelets, the component of blood that promotes clotting. Whenever you bleed, the platelets release serotonin to help constrict the blood vessels and minimize further loss of blood. The cells of your digestive tract also contain serotonin and serotonin receptors. The chemical regulates the secretion of stomach acid and other digestive fluids. It also stimulates certain intestinal muscles to contract, which helps move food along.

Our main concern, however, is with the role of serotonin within the brain. Serotonin influences a wide range of normal brain activity, including moods, eating patterns, pain transmission, sexual behavior, and sleep. The level of serotonin present in your brain can have a tremendous impact on how you think, feel, and behave. Having an adequate supply produces what is sometimes called the "serotonin effect"—a feeling of calmness, mild euphoria, and relaxation. Having too little serotonin can lead to the opposite situation—feelings of depression, anxiety, and other problems associated with serotonin deficiency syndrome (Table 1.1).

Table 1.1: The Effects of Different Levels of Serotonin

Optimal Level of Serotonin	*Low Level of Serotonin*
Hopeful, optimistic	Depressed
Calm	Anxious
Good-natured	Irritable
Patient	Impatient
Reflective and thoughtful	Impulsive
Loving and caring	Abusive
Able to concentrate	Short attention span
Creative, focused	Blocked, scattered
Able to think things through	Flies off the handle
Responsive	Reactive
Does not overeat carbohydrates	Craves sweets and high-carbohydrate foods
Sleeps well with good dream recall	Insomnia and poor dream recall

Out of the dozens of neurotransmitters, serotonin is the one most involved in the onset—and for that matter, the treatment—of various medical and psychiatric problems (Table 1.2). [If something goes wrong with the serotonin system, the impact can be tremendous. The consequences of serotonin deficiency syndrome can be devastating and include plunging moods, health-threatening food cravings, ruined sleep, skull-cracking headaches, overwhelming body pain, and just plain exhaustion. Because low serotonin can result from the stress and strain of our modern way of living, and because its symptoms severely reduce the joy of life to such a tremendous degree for so many people, I consider serotonin deficiency syndrome to be one of the most widespread and debilitating medical problems of our time.]

Table 1.2: Conditions Associated with Low Serotonin Levels

• Aggression
• Alcoholism

- Anxiety
- Attention deficit disorder
- Bulimia
- Carbohydrate cravings
- Chronic pain disorders (such as fibromyalgia)
- Depression
- Epilepsy
- Headaches (migraines, tension headaches, chronic headaches)
- Hyperactivity
- Insomnia
- Myoclonus (muscle twitching)
- Obesity
- Obsessive-compulsive disorder
- Panic disorders
- Premenstrual syndrome
- Schizophrenia
- Seasonal affective disorder ("winter depression")
- Suicidal thoughts and behavior

That serotonin is so deeply involved in so many brain functions comes as no surprise to scientists who study this complex organ. Research has shown that the activities of other types of neurotransmitters are concentrated in just a few areas of the brain. In contrast, clusters of serotonin-producing neurons are found in many key locations. For example, the part of the brain that controls our emotions—known as the limbic system—has a rich supply of serotonin neurons. The fibers branching out from serotonin-producing cells appear to be thicker and more densely woven into other parts of the brain than those of other neurons.

In recent years scientists have discovered that there are at least seven, and possibly as many as fifteen, subtypes of serotonin receptors. Each of these receptor types specializes in handling signals that govern different body functions. For example, one kind of serotonin receptor handles our response to anxiety, while another is in charge of blood vessel constriction.

The lower your level of serotonin, the more severe and widespread the potential impact on your brain and body. For example, low levels of serotonin can cause overwhelming sugar cravings. Research has shown that many people with bulimia, an eating disorder that causes uncontrollable eating binges, have insufficient supplies of serotonin. Low serotonin levels also are involved in depression, a common and often serious mental disorder characterized by very low mood and reduced levels of functioning. As you'll learn in more detail in the next chapter, a serious and life-threatening symptom of depression is suicidal thinking or, worse, suicidal behavior. Some scientific studies have found that people with the lowest levels of serotonin are at greatest risk of attempting—or committing—suicide. Lack of serotonin can disrupt your sleep patterns and lead to insomnia, as I'll explain in Chapter 4. Studies show that migraine headaches are the result of low serotonin levels and that boosting serotonin can prevent these headaches from developing (see Chapter 5). Because serotonin directly regulates the body's response to pain, and affects other neurotransmitters involved in pain control, maintaining adequate serotonin levels can relieve such pain syndromes as fibromyalgia, chronic fatigue syndrome, and premenstrual syndrome.

The problems arising from serotonin deficiency syndrome may vary from person to person. For example, in some people low levels of serotonin may cause depression, while in others the same level might produce regular disabling headaches or a voracious appetite for sweets and carbohydrates.

These variations in the effects of serotonin reflect human biochemical individuality. Although we all have the same basic electrochemical system in our brains, there are major differences in how we respond to the signals sent along that system in terms of mood and behavior.

The bottom line: If we hope to live a healthy, happy life, we need proper and balanced levels of key brain chemicals. But as I've said, the stress that results from our modern lifestyle can cause us to have insufficient levels of perhaps the most important of these chemicals, serotonin.

You might be wondering: If serotonin is so important, why can't I just increase my level by taking a pill or having an injection? The simple answer is that serotonin cannot safely be "imported" from the outside. It can only be manufactured *inside* the body, especially inside the brain. Like a factory, the brain needs an adequate supply of raw materials that it can modify to produce the final result: molecules of serotonin.

And the best source of that raw material—and one of the most exciting natural health breakthroughs of this or any decade—is 5-HTP.

Proteins

To understand why 5-HTP is unsurpassed for raising serotonin levels, you need to know a little more about how the body produces neurotransmitters. Here's the short version: [Brain chemicals are made from amino acids found in proteins that you consume in your diet. One of these amino acids is tryptophan. The conversion occurs in two key steps: First the body breaks down tryptophan to make 5-HTP, then it changes 5-HTP into serotonin.

That's the *Cliffs Notes* version. As you no doubt suspect, however, there's more to the story. Let's look at the process a little more closely.

Proteins are nutrients that are made of several different amino acids. You consume proteins in the foods you eat. During digestion, the protein molecule gets broken down into its component amino acids. The body then reassembles these amino acids into the dozens of other proteins it needs to function. That's why amino acids are often called the body's "building blocks."

The body must have at least twenty different kinds of amino acids to make the various proteins it needs to grow and function properly. But your body manufactures only twelve of these amino acids. The other eight, known as essential amino acids, must be consumed in the diet (Table 1.3).

Table 1.3: Amino Acids

Essential (from diet)	Nonessential (Endogenous)
Isoleucine	Alanine
Leucine	Arginine
Lysine	Aspartic acid
Methionine	Cysteine
Phenylalanine	Glutamic acid
Threonine	Glutamine
Tryptophan	Glycine
Valine	Histidine
	Hydroxyproline
	Proline
	Serine
	Tyrosine

Your body uses certain proteins (known as fibrous proteins) to create tissues such as skin, hair, nails, muscles, and tendons. Proteins linked with molecules of fat form the membranes that hold individual cells together. Another kind (the globular proteins) are the basis for neurotransmitters, hormones, enzymes, and the substances that form the body's immune response against infection. Some amino acids are broken down into still smaller pieces to form DNA, the genetic material found inside your cells. As you can see, proteins are absolutely vital for a healthy, functioning body.

Not all proteins are created equal. Some proteins provide certain types of amino acids, while other proteins provide different kinds. That's why it's important that you eat a varied diet, since no single food contains all the ingredients your body needs. A complete protein is one that contains all eight of the essential amino acids (that is, the ones your body can't manufacture). Foods that provide high levels of complete protein include meat, poultry, fish, eggs, milk, and cheese. Nuts and legumes (peas and beans) contain some but not all of the essential amino acids; these are known as incomplete proteins. Vegetarians—people who do not eat meat—must plan their diets carefully to make sure they eat the right combination of vegetables, fruits, and grains needed to supply all the various kinds of essential amino acids.

The amino acid that we are most interested in here is called tryptophan (pronounced TRIP-toh-fan). The body changes tryptophan into serotonin through a series of steps. Because tryptophan is an essential amino acid, we must consume an adequate supply in our diet. Good sources of tryptophan include milk, cottage cheese, poultry (turkey and chicken), eggs, red meats, soybeans, tofu, and nuts, especially almonds.

Until recently in the United States, tryptophan was also available over the counter as a dietary supplement. Because of the medical problems caused by contaminated supplies of tryptophan (which I'll explain in a moment), it is now available only by prescription. Fortunately, there's a better way to boost serotonin levels, and that's by taking 5-HTP. To understand 5-HTP's recent meteoric rise to prominence, let's look at what happened to tryptophan a few years ago.

The L-Tryptophan Crisis: A Bit of History

The importance of serotonin in maintaining physical and emotional health has been known for decades. Because the body makes serotonin from tryptophan, it is possible to take doses of dietary supplements containing L-tryptophan to raise serotonin levels. (In this book I use the word *tryptophan* to mean the amino acid found naturally in food, and the term *L-tryptophan* to refer specifically to the amino acid manufactured for commercial use in pill or powder form.) In the United States alone, for more than three decades, L-tryptophan was used by more than thirty million people as an effective treatment for insomnia, depression, over-eating, and a range of other problems.

However, in October of 1989, some people taking L-tryptophan began experiencing troubling symptoms: severe muscle and joint pain (myalgia), high fever, weakness, swelling in the arms and legs, and shortness of breath. Tests found that these people had very high levels of a kind of white blood cell known as eosinophils. Usually eosinophil levels rise when the body mounts an immune response to fight off allergy attacks or parasitic infections. Research soon showed, however, that this group of symptoms—which became known as eosinophilia-myalgia syndrome, or EMS—developed in people who did not have such medical problems. The only thing victims of EMS had in common was that they were all taking L-tryptophan supplements. Eventually over fifteen hundred cases of EMS were reported in the United States. Nearly thirty people died in the first year of the epidemic, and to date over fifty people have died from the illness.[2]

As a result of the problem, the Food and Drug Administration asked manufacturers and distributors to voluntarily recall L-tryptophan. At the time this book is being written, the recall remains in effect and is likely to continue for the foreseeable future. As a result, you can no longer walk into a health food store and buy a bottle of L-tryptophan. However, L-tryptophan is available by prescription, and it is still approved for use as an ingredient in infant formulas and nutrient mixtures used in hospitals for intravenous feedings.

To find out what caused the problem, several teams of scientists, including a group at the Centers for Disease Control (CDC) led by Edwin M. Kilbourne, examined all the available evidence. They concluded that the cause of the EMS epidemic could be traced to batches of L-tryptophan that were produced between October 1988 and July 1989 by a single manufacturer in Japan, a company called Showa Denko.[3] The largest of six Japanese makers of L-tryptophan, Showa Denko had supplied between 50 percent and 60 percent of all the L-tryptophan sold in the United States. The company made L-tryptophan by a process that involved fermentation using a type of bacteria, a common method of producing certain kinds of drugs and other chemicals.

The problem was not with L-tryptophan itself, or even with its use as a dietary supplement. Instead, the researchers discovered that the L-tryptophan had become contaminated due to changes the company had made in its fermentation and filtering processes.[4] As serious as the epidemic was, it could have been worse; the chances that a person who took contaminated L-tryptophan made by Showa Denko would develop EMS were 1 in 250.[5]

The FDA acted responsibly in taking steps to protect the public from a dangerous, even fatal, hazard until the cause could be identified. In the future, the agency may decide to end the voluntary recall and allow the sale of L-tryptophan in over-the-counter products. Meanwhile, L-tryptophan continues to be widely used as an approved treatment for depression, insomnia, and other conditions in Italy, Spain, France, Germany, and other countries. Strict new guidelines have been implemented to ensure the purity and safety of L-tryptophan.[6] It is important to emphasize that no cases of EMS have ever been traced to use of *un*contaminated L-tryptophan.[7]

One very positive development arising from the EMS crisis was that it led to a search for a nonprescription alternative to L-tryptophan, one that provides all the serotonin-boosting benefits of tryptophan at lower doses and without risk. That alternative is 5-HTP.

Tryptophan to 5-HTP to Serotonin

The process by which your body produces serotonin from tryptophan is both intricate and fascinating. By understanding the process, you'll realize that 5-HTP is one step closer to serotonin in the body than tryptophan is. Taking 5-HTP thus gives your body a jump start in its efforts to maintain healthy levels of serotonin.

To release the tryptophan (and other nutrients) from the food you eat, the food particles must first be digested, or broken down into smaller pieces. Digestion begins as soon as food comes into contact with the saliva in your mouth. Saliva contains enzymes, which, as I noted earlier, work by snipping large molecules into smaller units. Other enzymes and fluids inside your stomach continue the process of digestion.

Eventually the digested food—now called *chyme* (pronounced "kime")—passes into the small intestine. The intestine is lined with thousands of tiny, soft, fingerlike projections called *villi* (plural of the word *villus*). Under the microscope, the villi look like the fibers on a carpet. The villi absorb the nutrients from the chyme as it flows past. Absorption is the next crucial step in *metabolism,* a general term that refers to all the chemical processes taking place in your body.

Tryptophan molecules (and other chemicals) then pass from the villi into the bloodstream. The blood carries tryptophan to different parts of the body, where the process of conversion continues. Some conversion happens in tissues such as the digestive system. But the main activity occurs in the liver and in the brain. Let's discuss what happens in the liver first.

The amount of tryptophan that changes into 5-HTP inside the liver depends on the body's other metabolic needs at that moment. Once tryptophan arrives in the liver, one of four things can happen:

✓ • The tryptophan can pass, unchanged, directly back into the blood to be used elsewhere in the body.

- Certain liver enzymes can get to work cutting the tryptophan into other, smaller proteins needed for healthy blood.
- An enzyme called tryptophan hydrolase can convert tryptophan into molecules of 5-HTP. Since our goal is to raise serotonin levels, that's what we want to happen.
- Tryptophan gets changed into another substance called *kynurenine* (pronounced kine-YUR-uh-nin).

Let's talk a little more about kynurenine, which is made when an enzyme called tryptophan oxygenase comes into contact with the tryptophan molecule. Kynurenine is a convulsant, which means it works as a potent muscle stimulant. Your body needs a certain amount of kynurenine to function properly. But if the levels of kynurenine get too high, there is a risk of muscle damage. Over time, this damage may lead to chronic conditions such as Parkinson's disease. Generally, in the liver, more tryptophan is converted to kynurenine than to 5-HTP. For that reason, trying to regulate serotonin by taking supplemental L-tryptophan may increase the risk of muscle disorders, because it raises your kynurenine levels. I'm talking here only about the use of supplements; the amount of tryptophan contained in a normal diet does not pose this risk. What's more, since 5-HTP is already a converted form of tryptophan, taking doses of 5-HTP does not lead to increased kynurenine levels.

Other factors can also affect the rate at which the liver converts tryptophan into kynurenine or other substances. Stress, for example, can increase kynurenine production because it reduces the supply of the important enzyme tryptophan hydrolase, needed to change tryptophan into 5-HTP. As I noted at the beginning of this chapter, stress takes many forms: emotional upheaval, physical illness, or pressure from work or other daily activities. When your body is under stress, it reacts by releasing other hormones to protect you from the damage stress causes. One such hormone is cortisol, which counteracts inflammation. When your cortisol levels are high, your liver releases *more* of the enzyme that con-

verts tryptophan into kynurenine and *less* of the enzyme you need
to make 5-HTP. If your tryptophan supply is used up in making
kynurenine, then there will be less available to make 5-HTP (and
thus, ultimately, serotonin).

Other factors that inhibit or reduce the rate of conversion to
5-HTP include low levels of B vitamins (especially vitamin B_6 and
niacin), low magnesium levels, insensitivity to insulin, and genetic
deficiencies.

As you can see, the liver is one of the main "factories" for
5-HTP. But the process doesn't end there. Molecules of 5-HTP
must then pass back into the bloodstream so they can travel to the
brain, where they will be converted into serotonin. Ultimately,
then, the level of serotonin in your brain depends to a large extent
on what happens to tryptophan in the liver. If the tryptophan
changes to kynurenine, it will never become serotonin. Nor will
most of the tryptophan that is used to make blood proteins. However, unchanged tryptophan that passes into the bloodstream may
yet be converted to serotonin in the brain. So too may 5-HTP.

But that won't happen unless and until those molecules can
enter the brain.

Kynurenine
5 HTP

5-HTP and the Blood-Brain Barrier

To carry out its many vital functions, the brain needs vast
amounts of energy and nourishment. At any given time, approximately 15 percent of your body's entire blood supply is flowing
through your brain. To handle this flow, the brain is laced by a
complex network of blood vessels, the smallest of which are called
capillaries.

Capillaries in the brain are different from those found in the
rest of your body. Most capillaries in the body have a "wall" or
membrane that contains numerous small openings (Figure 1.3).
These openings exist between cells of the membrane, like gates
positioned between segments of a brick wall. The openings allow

molecules of various sizes to leave the bloodstream easily and pass into the surrounding fluid. This is how nutrients and other substances, such as medicines, pass out of the bloodstream so they can enter the cells and do their work.

But the brain is so important to the body that it has to be protected from the presence of unwanted chemicals that might disrupt its function. To block passage of these chemicals, the membranes of the capillaries in the brain do not have the openings found in capillaries located elsewhere in the body. Instead the membranes are made of tightly overlapping cells with no openings. These are called *glial cells; glia* is the same Greek word from which we get our word *glue*. Like glue, these cells help hold the membrane together and prohibit passage of certain molecules. Glial cells contain high levels of fatty molecules called *lipids*.

In a sense, these capillary membranes act like the security clearance desks in top-level government buildings. If a molecule wants to leave the capillary and enter the brain, it can't simply flow through a hole in the membrane, as it can elsewhere in the body. Instead it must first merge with and pass directly through the surface of one of the glial cells. Basically, what happens is that the molecule grabs onto the fatty part of the glial cell. Molecules that can do so easily are called *lipid-soluble*. The molecule can only bind with this fatty part and pass through if it has the right ID—that is, the right combination of properties. If the molecules are not very lipid-soluble, if they are too large or have the wrong shape, or if they contain potentially poisonous compounds, the glial cells of the membrane will block their passage. This life-saving protective system is known as the blood-brain barrier.

The blood-brain barrier is effective at its job—sometimes almost too effective. Like an overzealous security guard, the barrier can also make it difficult for certain "authorized" molecules to gain entry to the brain. Sometimes, for example, vital nutrients from food or the active ingredients in medications might be denied access, at least temporarily.

The fact that the blood-brain barrier is so selective in what it

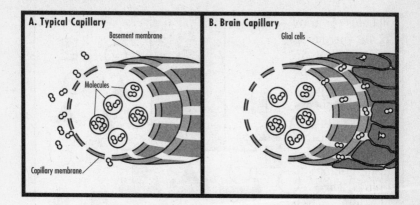

Figure 1.3: The Blood-Brain Barrier

allows to enter the brain is another important part of the 5-HTP story. Both tryptophan and 5-HTP have "clearance" to permeate the barrier—but their levels of clearance are different. Before tryptophan can pass through, it first must have an escort. The tryptophan molecule must attach itself to a certain protein, called a *transport molecule,* found on the surface of the membrane cells. Once it binds to the transport molecule, tryptophan attains the necessary "clearance" to pass through the capillary membrane and enter the brain. However, only limited numbers of these transport molecules are available, and they are needed to transport not just tryptophan but all the other amino acids as well. If these transport molecules are busy serving other "visitors," then tryptophan molecules have to wait their turn until an escort becomes available.

How long tryptophan must wait before entering the brain depends on various factors. The main issue is the balance of other amino acids in the bloodstream, which in turn is determined by the types of foods in your diet. Compared to other amino acids, tryptophan is found in foods only in small quantities. A few hours after you eat a high-protein meal, such as one containing meat, there will be high levels of many different amino acids, all com-

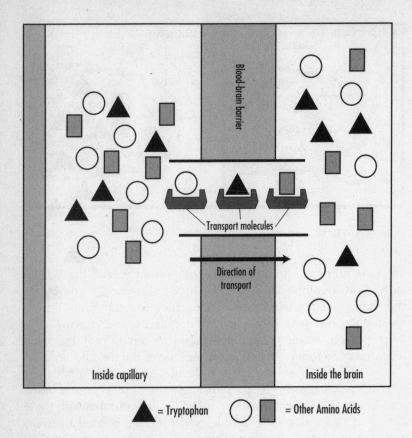

Figure 1.4A: Transport Across the Blood-Brain Barrier.

peting for a ride into the brain on the few available transport molecules (Figure 1.4A). On the other hand, if you eat a high-carbohydrate meal, then there will be relatively higher levels of tryptophan and lower levels of other amino acids. In that case, tryptophan enters the brain more quickly, and the level of serotonin rises (Figure 1.4B).

But 5-HTP is different—and in that difference lies the key to 5-HTP's superiority over tryptophan as a way of boosting seroto-

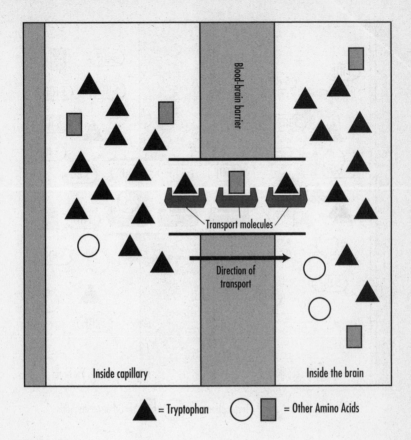

Figure 1.4B

nin. Because the stripped-down 5-HTP molecule is more lipid-soluble than tryptophan and is already closer in structure to serotonin inside the brain, it has a higher level of "security clearance." That means it doesn't need to wait for a transport molecule to become available before it can pass through the capillary membrane. As soon as a 5-HTP molecule shows up at the blood-brain barrier, it is admitted to the brain, like a first-class passenger on an airline (Figure 1.4C).

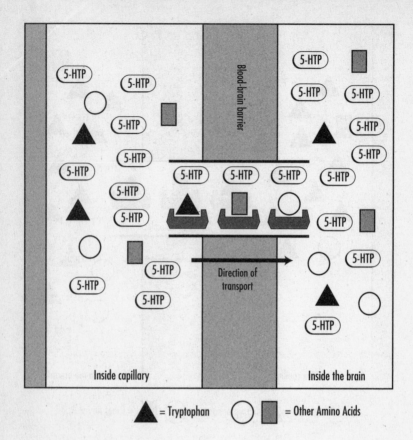

Figure 1.4C

Once inside the brain, 5-HTP is available for conversion to serotonin. The final conversion process requires another few steps and involves the activity of a series of enzymes, which I won't detail here. Suffice it to say that everything has to work properly for you to achieve the proper serotonin levels.

Eventually, though, the tryptophan that you consumed in your meal—or that dose of 5-HTP you took twenty minutes ago or so—gets processed into its final form: the powerful and important neurotransmitter serotonin.

5-HTP vs. Tryptophan: A Comparison

The crisis that resulted from contaminated supplies of L-tryptophan proved to be a blessing in disguise because it shifted the spotlight to 5-HTP as an alternative way to boost serotonin levels. Research has shown that, by all measures, 5-HTP is far superior to either tryptophan or L-tryptophan. Here are some of the reasons why:

- Commercially available 5-HTP that has been extracted from a natural source, the seed of an African plant known as *Griffonia simplicifolia,* is not vulnerable to contamination. One process by which L-tryptophan is manufactured involves fermentation using bacteria, which does pose a risk of contamination.
- 5-HTP, unlike both tryptophan and L-tryptophan, cannot be metabolized by the liver into kynurenine. In fact, the higher the dose of L-tryptophan, the more kynurenine produced. Once that conversion happens, kynurenine cannot then be converted into serotonin. In contrast, none of the dose of 5-HTP is lost by conversion into kynurenine.
- While about 70 percent of a dose of 5-HTP taken orally is delivered to the bloodstream for transport to the brain,[8] only about 3 percent of a dose of L-tryptophan is eventually converted into serotonin.[9]
- 5-HTP passes into the brain immediately, while tryp-

tophan must compete with other proteins to be transported across the blood-brain barrier.

- 5-HTP raises levels of other brain neurotransmitters, including melatonin, dopamine, and norepinephrine. L-tryptophan does not have this effect.
- Some people have a genetic defect that prevents their bodies from converting tryptophan to 5-HTP efficiently. Taking 5-HTP bypasses this step, however, and overcomes the genetic problem.
- 5-HTP has been found to exert significant protection against free-radical formation and oxidative damage. In contrast, high doses of L-tryptophan may promote the formation of free radicals.

SUGAR, SLEEP, AND SEROTONIN

Have you ever noticed that you get a little sleepy after you eat meals that contain lots of starches or sugars? There's a good reason for that. To metabolize carbohydrates, your body releases high levels of a hormone called insulin. Insulin's primary job is to remove sugar from the blood and help it pass into the cells, where it can be burned for energy. At the same time, insulin promotes the absorption into tissues of various amino acids. After a high-carbohydrate meal, there are fewer molecules of amino acids circulating in the bloodstream. As a result, there are fewer amino acids to compete with tryptophan for transport through the blood-brain barrier. Tryptophan thus gets priority for admission. The same thing happens if you eat foods rich in tryptophan, such as turkey, or if you take doses of 5-HTP. With higher levels of tryptophan or 5-HTP available, the brain can manufacture more serotonin. One function of serotonin is to help you feel calm and relaxed. That's why many people get drowsy two or three hours after eating a carbohydrate-rich or tryptophan-packed meal. No wonder we often feel like nodding off after a big traditional Thanksgiving dinner!

As I'll discuss in Chapter 4, 5-HTP is a very valuable method of treating sleep disorders such as insomnia. Taken in the right doses and throughout the day, it improves sleep quality without causing daytime drowsiness.

5-HTP as an Antioxidant

Among the most exciting aspects of 5-HTP is its potential role in protecting the body against free radicals. Briefly defined, a free radical is an unstable molecule, a tiny loose cannon that can do enormous damage to cells and tissues.

A quick chemistry lesson: All molecules contain small particles called electrons. Normally electrons come in pairs. However, when your body burns oxygen molecules to supply your cells with energy, one of the electrons in a pair can sometimes get stripped away. For electrons, being alone in the world violates the most fundamental laws of nature. As a result, any oxygen molecule with an unpaired electron goes on a frantic search to find another electron to complete its set. Like a determined mother questing for the newest Beanie Baby, the molecule will latch on to any available electron it can find—including one that is already being used by another molecule. In the process of "stealing" this electron, however, the free radical can ruthlessly destroy the other molecule. The resulting damage is known as oxidation. To get a sense of what oxidation does to the body, picture what happens to a slice of apple when it is exposed to the air for a few minutes. Oxidation is what causes the brown spots to appear.

To a large extent, the aging process is a result of damage by free radicals. These lethal molecules are also involved as underlying causes of two of the biggest killers in the United States, heart disease and cancer.

But the body doesn't take assault by free radicals lying down. It sends in the cavalry—in the form of antioxidants—to "mop up" the marauding molecules. Types of antioxidants include vitamin C, beta-carotene, selenium, and vitamin E.

And lately another powerful antioxidant has been added to the list. A study conducted at the United States National Center for Radiation Research found that 5-HTP exerts significant protection against free-radical formation and oxidative damage. In contrast, L-tryptophan—the commercial form of tryptophan—offered no antioxidant activity. Quite the opposite: In high doses, dietary tryptophan or L-tryptophan may actually *increase* the rate at which free radicals form.[10]

Thus, in addition to its potential role in treating a range of conditions from depression to insomnia, taking 5-HTP may help slow down the aging process and protect the body against serious—and potentially fatal—illnesses.[11] Research in this area is just beginning. We need a lot more studies to fully understand 5-HTP's role as a potential antioxidant. But no doubt we will see some exciting developments in the near future.

5-HTP and Other Neurotransmitter Systems

5-HTP AND MELATONIN

As you have seen, the process by which your body makes serotonin is intricate and complex. But the process doesn't end with serotonin. In fact, serotonin is the "parent molecule" your brain needs to make another vital hormone called melatonin.

You have probably heard about melatonin. It became a hot

topic a few years ago when people learned about its health-related properties. Now widely available as a nutritional supplement, melatonin is used to treat insomnia, jet lag, stress, and depression. Although studies are not yet complete, there is preliminary evidence suggesting that melatonin may also reduce the risk of heart disease by lowering cholesterol, reducing high blood pressure, and preventing clots from forming in blood vessels. Because melatonin may act as an antioxidant, there is some hope that this hormone may even help prevent cancer.

Melatonin is released by the *pineal* (py-NEE-ul) gland. This tiny, cone-shaped clump of tissue is located at the very center of your brain. The level of melatonin secretion changes over the course of a day, with most of the melatonin being released at night.

Because your body uses 5-HTP to make serotonin, and because serotonin is used to make melatonin, taking 5-HTP may help you achieve the benefits of melatonin. More information about this subject appears in Chapter 4.

5-HTP AND ENDORPHINS

As I mentioned earlier, endorphins are neuropeptides, neurotransmitters made from chains of two or more amino acids. Endorphins, which are chemically related to morphine, are the body's own pain relievers.

The role of endorphins in the body first came to light during the jogging craze a few decades ago. Runners who took part in marathons noticed that after running for several miles, the pain of their exertion was replaced by a flood of good feeling—the so-called runner's high. Scientists soon learned that this sensation of euphoria resulted when the body secreted higher levels of certain pain-easing molecules, which they called endorphins.

The name combines two medical terms, *endo-* (meaning "within") and *morphine.* Morphine, named after Morpheus, the

Roman god of dreams, is a powerful pain-relieving drug derived from the opium poppy plant. Morphine works by blocking the transmission of pain signals at specific sites (called opiate receptors) in the brain and spinal cord, thereby preventing the perception of pain. It also induces a general feeling of relaxation and well-being. Like morphine, molecules of endorphin also bind to the opiate receptors and block pain signals from traveling along the nerves. The most important of these neurotransmitters is known as beta-endorphin.

Pain sensations are a vital part of your body's functioning. You need to be able to feel pain as a warning signal that something is wrong. (If you didn't flinch with pain when you put your hand on a hot stove, you might suffer severe burns and permanent damage.) But too much pain lasting for too long a period can also be debilitating. Nature thus provides your body with endorphins as a built-in mechanism for damping, but not eliminating, pain.

If you get sick, or if you suffer from stress or experience an emotional upset, your body releases endorphins. But the supply is limited. If the condition persists for a long time, you can exhaust your supply. Laboratory tests show that people who have chronic complaints such as stress, depression, chronic fatigue syndrome, and fibromyalgia (a condition that causes chronic overall muscle and joint pain) have low levels of endorphins.

Fortunately, there is a way to restore your endorphin supply. Mounting evidence suggests that taking 5-HTP can boost endorphin levels. This is because 5-HTP increases serotonin, and serotonin, in its role as "master molecule," regulates the production and release of endorphins. Although we are focusing in this book on serotonin as the star of the neurotransmitter system, beta-endorphins probably qualify for second billing. A comparison of the effects of high and low levels of endorphins reveals the profound impact these chemicals have on our feelings and behavior (Table 1.4).

Table 1.4: The Effects of Different Levels
of Beta-Endorphin

Optimal Level of Beta-Endorphin	*Low Level of Beta-Endorphin*
High tolerance for pain	Low pain tolerance
Sensitive, sympathetic	Tearful, reactive
High self-esteem	Low self-esteem
Compassionate	Overwhelmed by others' pain
Connected and in touch	Feels isolated
Hopeful, optimistic, euphoric	Depressed, hopeless
Takes personal responsibility	Feels like a victim
Solution-oriented	Emotionally overwhelmed
No addiction to sweet foods	Craves sweets

5-HTP AND OTHER NEUROTRANSMITTERS

To function at its peak, and to maintain mood, the brain needs a good balance in the supply and activity of all the neurotransmitters. Besides its effects on the melatonin and the endorphin systems, 5-HTP has been shown to raise levels of other brain neurotransmitters, including dopamine and norepinephrine.[12] The ability of 5-HTP to affect the brain chemicals in the indoleamine family as well as their cousins the catecholamines helps explain why it has such a broad spectrum of effects throughout the body.

Summary

We need adequate levels of serotonin to function at our best— to stay active, alert, well rested, and happy. Low levels of serotonin can lead to depression, sleep problems, eating disorders, pain syndromes, and a number of other complications. Taking 5-HTP gives the body the metabolic boost it needs to manufacture serotonin safely and effectively, and to fight back against serotonin deficiency syndrome.

Key Points in This Chapter

- Serotonin is a neurotransmitter that is vital for optimal brain function.
- Serotonin deficiency syndrome is linked to a number of serious health problems, including obesity, depression, insomnia, pain syndromes, and headaches.
- It is possible to raise serotonin levels by increasing intake of tryptophan in the diet or by taking tryptophan supplements (L-tryptophan), although tryptophan as a supplement is no longer available in the United States without a prescription.
- 5-HTP is a well-researched, natural way to boost serotonin levels and treat conditions linked to low serotonin. It is safer and more effective than L-tryptophan.
- 5-HTP increases the supply and enhances the activity of other neurotransmitters, including melatonin and the endorphins.
- 5-HTP acts as an antioxidant, which means it may prevent aging-related damage to the body and may reduce the risk of serious diseases such as cancer.

CHAPTER 2

5-HTP AND DEPRESSION

To judge by appearances, you'd have thought Linda had everything going for her. An attractive brunette, she was just a few months shy of her twenty-first birthday. She was earning high marks at college, which she was attending on a music scholarship for the study of classical piano. She had been dating a classmate pretty steadily for the past few months and they were even beginning to talk about getting married.

But clearly something was wrong. When Linda spoke, her words trickled out in a slow monotone. Her mouth never registered more than the faintest and most flickering of smiles. And her eyes were puffy and glazed.

Linda had come to see me because she was worried that her flagging energy would jeopardize her ability to get through the grueling final exam period just a few weeks away. She was struggling to concentrate on her studies but was barely able to read more than a page of her textbooks before her mind would start wandering. Before, she had been able to zip through a tricky Bach fugue without batting an eye. But now, she said, the notes on the page looked like unintelligible hieroglyphics and her once-responsive fingers failed to obey her commands. She had been guzzling coffee and high-caffeine sodas, she said, to try to jump-start her system. Yes, she said, she was getting enough sleep—from nine to eleven hours a night—but still she woke up feeling sluggish and unrefreshed.

I asked how long this had been going on.

"Six weeks, maybe," she replied. "Maybe longer—a couple of months."

Then I asked a key question, one that I ask all my patients: "What is it that gives you pleasure in your life?"

The pause before Linda answered seemed agonizingly long. Finally her lips parted and she muttered, "Nothing."

Here was a young woman with brains, beauty, talent, and love. She should have been savoring her present and looking forward to a bright and fulfilling future. Instead she seemed sunk in a swamp of sadness and self-pity. The music in her soul was dying.

I gave Linda a physical exam and conducted blood tests to see if a physical disease might be causing her emotional tailspin, but I found nothing. On the line for diagnosis in Linda's chart, I wrote *depression.*

Darkness Visible

Depression is a such a widespread problem that some experts have called it the "common cold" of psychiatric disorders. Each year a staggering number of Americans—over fifteen million—suffer from this debilitating condition. In 1996 over twenty-eight million people in this country—one in every ten—were taking a prescription antidepressant medication.

Despite its prevalence, depression is still not very well understood. Often people say they are depressed when they experience a minor disappointment or temporary loss. But true depression—what doctors call clinical depression—is not the same as feeling a little blue or "down in the dumps" for a day or two. Instead it is a serious illness with potentially tragic consequences. The noted author William Styron, author of *Sophie's Choice,* described his depression as "darkness visible." As my patient Linda found, depression can diminish people's spark, their drive, their zest for life. Tragically, in some cases depression can rob them of life itself.

Why are so many people depressed? A substantial body of scientific evidence shows that depression results from disturbances in the brain's chemical system. The main problem arises with imbalances or other defects involving the neurotransmitters. As you learned in Chapter 1, these include the monoamines melatonin, dopamine, and norepinephrine. More specifically, depression often arises as a consequence of the serotonin deficiency syndrome.

Since the 1950s, doctors have treated depression by prescribing medications that tinker with the brain's neurotransmitter system. The advent of Prozac in the late 1980s marked a giant step forward. As I'll explain in more detail later in this chapter, Prozac works by preventing the reabsorption (or reuptake) of serotonin by the brain cells (Figure 2.1). This means that serotonin remains in circulation in the gaps between the cells, which allows your brain to make maximum use of its available supply of serotonin. As a result, it is better able to carry out its normal functions, such as regulating mood, appetite, and sleep.

What's more, Prozac and its chemical cousins seem to affect *only* serotonin. They do not interfere with the activity of other neurotransmitter systems. For that reason, scientists classify these drugs, including Zoloft and Paxil, as *selective serotonin reuptake inhibitors*, or SSRIs for short.

The SSRIs have helped millions of people overcome their depression. They also appear to relieve a number of other related conditions, including anxiety and obsessive-compulsive disorder.

As effective as they are, however, the SSRIs have some serious drawbacks. For one thing, although they prevent the reuptake of serotonin, they do nothing to increase the brain's basic supply of the neurotransmitter. Thus they may be of little benefit to people

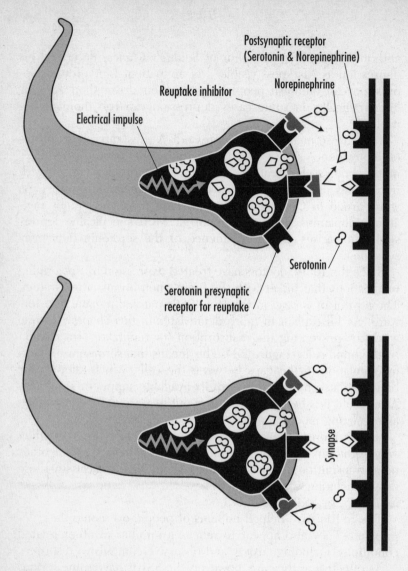

Figure 2.1: Reuptake

whose bodies do not produce adequate levels of serotonin. At the same time, SSRIs can cause a number of serious side effects, including nausea, fatigue, agitation, and a loss of interest in sex.

As I'll explain in this chapter, 5-HTP is a safe and effective natural alternative to the SSRIs for addressing depression, one of the most serious manifestations of the serotonin deficiency syndrome. When used as part of a comprehensive program that also promotes lifestyle modifications in such areas as diet, exercise, and stress management, 5-HTP can help lift moods, improve sleep, and restore the sense of pleasure in simply being alive.

Depression Defined

Doctors use the term "clinical depression" to indicate that the condition is serious enough to require treatment. One problem in dealing with depression is that the definition is somewhat broad. The list of symptoms is long, and the disorder can affect different people in different ways. My patient Linda, for example, would sleep long hours but would awaken groggy and unrefreshed. Paradoxically, however, most people with depression tend to wake up early and then find themselves unable to fall back asleep.

In fact, depression is not a single illness but a spectrum of conditions ranging from mild to severe, even life-threatening. Let's take a quick look at the different types of depression.

UNIPOLAR (MAJOR) DEPRESSION

According to the official guidebook of the American Psychiatric Association, the *Diagnostic and Statistical Manual of Mental Disorders—Fourth Edition* (DSM-IV), clinical depression involves some combination of the following main characteristics:[1]

- Appetite changes (increase or decrease), especially when such changes lead to weight loss or gain

- Changes in sleep patterns
  - Insomnia (inability to fall asleep or, more commonly, waking too early in the morning and being unable to fall back asleep)
  - Hypersomnia (wanting to sleep all of the time)
- Physical inactivity and sluggishness (or, paradoxically, hyperactivity)
- Decreased interest or pleasure in usual activities, such as lowered sexual drive, withdrawal from friends and family, loss of interest in work or hobbies
- Loss of energy and feelings of fatigue
- Feelings of worthlessness, self-reproach, inappropriate guilt, and hopelessness about the future
- Diminished ability to think or concentrate
- Recurrent thoughts of death or suicide, or actual suicidal behavior

According to the DSM-IV definition, the presence of five of these features for a period of at least four weeks is a clear sign of major depression. Another term for this condition is *unipolar depression.* "Unipolar" means that the person's mood swings in one direction: downward. The mood might return to normal after a while, either on its own or in response to treatment. Some people experience only one episode of major depression, although that episode might last for months, even years. Many others, however, experience repeated bouts of major depression throughout their lives. This condition is known as recurrent depression.

Linda, the patient we met at the beginning of this chapter, was experiencing an episode of major depression. Her mood, activity level, and ability to concentrate had all bottomed out. She was sleeping far too much for a young woman enrolled in a demanding course of study, yet her sleep was of very poor quality. Although it seemed she had everything going for her, she was unable to identify any sources of joy or delight in her life. She needed help, and I suggested that 5-HTP was the answer.

DYSTHYMIA

Mild depression is also known as *dysthymia*. (The Greek term *thym-* means "mood.") In previous decades, dysthymia was known by various names, including depressive personality and depressive neurosis, although these terms carry far more stigma than *dysthymia*. The condition afflicts millions of people in the United States alone.

Although it is generally a mild disorder, dysthymia can nonetheless drain the juice out of a person's life. Fortunately, it is a medical condition that responds well to appropriate treatment. According to the DSM-IV criteria, a patient must be depressed most of the time for at least two years (one year for children or adolescents) to qualify for a diagnosis of dysthymia. In addition, at least three of the following symptoms must be present:

- Low self-esteem or lack of self-confidence
- Pessimism, hopelessness, or despair
- Lack of interest in ordinary pleasures and activities
- Withdrawal from social activities
- Fatigue or lethargy
- Guilt or ruminating about the past
- Irritability or excessive anger
- Diminished productivity
- Difficulty concentrating or making decisions

BIPOLAR DISORDER (MANIC-DEPRESSION) AND HYPOMANIA

In contrast to unipolar depression, *bipolar depression* involves dramatic mood swings from deep, despairing lows to frantic, frenzied highs. A person suffering from a bipolar mood disorder might be laughing, buoyant, and energetic one day, and hopeless, despairing, even suicidal the next. Some people experience such mood changes over the course of a few days, but in other cases the changes can occur very quickly, even within a matter of minutes. Such cases are known as "rapid cycling bipolar disorder." Some people experience elevated moods that don't quite reach the level of full-fledged mania; this condition is called *hypomania.* (*Hypo-* means "low" or "beneath.")

According to the DSM-IV, a diagnosis of bipolar mood disorder involves at least three of the following symptoms:

- Excessive self-esteem or grandiosity (feelings of self-importance or omnipotence)
- Reduced need for sleep or going for several days without sleep
- Extreme talkativeness (for example, excessive telephoning)
- Extremely rapid flight of thoughts along with the feeling that the mind is racing
- Inability to concentrate, easily distracted
- Increase in social or work-oriented activities, such as a frantic eighty-hour work week
- Poor judgment, as indicated by sprees of uncontrolled spending, increased sexual indiscretions, or misguided financial decisions

People in the throes of a full-blown manic attack usually need to be hospitalized. During manic episodes, people may lose control; they may hurt themselves or others, or engage in potentially destructive activities such as spending all their money or launching impossible business schemes.

Dispelling the Black Cloud:

HELEN'S STORY

Something in the tone of the voice I heard on my voice mail sent a chill up my spine. The woman, who identified herself as Helen, sounded desperate. She said she had read my book *Natural Alternatives to Prozac* and wanted to see me. "I was on Prozac and it just about sent me over the edge," she said. "I really need help." I called her back and told her to come to my office as soon as she could.

To put it bluntly, Helen was a mess. This thirty-three-year-old divorced mother of two had struggled with depression for years. The battle had taken its toll: Her face was pale, her appearance untidy. Her whole body seemed to be dragged down, as if the pull of gravity was stronger wherever she was standing.

"I feel like that character in the *Li'l Abner* comic strip, the one who always had that black rain cloud hanging over his head," she said.

Helen had been hospitalized twice in the course of the previous year for depression. After the first stay in the hospital, she was discharged with a prescription for Prozac. "It made me nuts," she said. When I pressed her for more details, she said that within a few days after she started taking the medication she got very agitated—"real hyper," as she put it. One afternoon her younger child started drawing on the wall with a laundry marker. "I just snapped," Helen recalled with a shudder. She described how she went on a rampage, tearing up the room, smashing furniture and light fixtures, whacking holes in the wall with a meat mallet. When she realized what she had done—and how close she had come to harming her child—she ran into the bathroom and swallowed the entire contents of a bottle of aspirin. "I didn't care if I lived or died," she said. Her older daughter, age seven, had the presence of mind to call 911, and Helen was taken to the hospital.

Helen was one of those people in whom an antidepressant produces a very dangerous condition known as *akathisia*—a drug-induced state of agitation. Soon after Prozac came on the market, several reports appeared stating that the drug could trigger violent, even suicidal behavior. The link between Prozac and violence or suicide is highly controversial. Some studies have found a connection,[2] while others have not.[3] The final verdict is not yet in, but because of my experience with patients like Helen, I continue to be convinced that we should seek natural alternatives to these potent and potentially dangerous drugs whenever possible.

I did an extensive workup on Helen and suggested that she try taking 5-HTP at a relatively high dosage: 150 mg three times a day. I also prescribed St.-John's-wort extract, 300 mg per day, to boost the effects of the 5-HTP. (For more information, see Chapter 7). I gave Helen strict instructions to call me each day to tell me how she was doing.

I admit that although I am a firm believer in the value of 5-HTP, I wasn't prepared for the results. Helen called every day, as promised. For the first four days things stayed pretty much the same. But on the fifth day the contrast was startling. "I can't believe it," Helen said. "I woke up today feeling happy. That's the first time in years." I was a little suspicious, and I worried that she might have been exaggerating her response just to please me. But over the days and weeks that followed, it was clear that something had changed for Helen in a profound way. She felt calmer, more in control. She no longer felt those violent urges, and she expressed amazement that she had ever thought about killing herself at all.

It's been about six months since I first met Helen. In that time I reduced her daily regimen to 100 mg of 5-HTP plus 300 mg of St.-John's-wort extract taken at bedtime. She appears to be doing fine. "I have my down days," she told me recently. "Who doesn't? Raising two kids on your own is not always a picnic. But at least I don't see that black cloud looming overhead anymore."

5-HTP and the Treatment of Depression

The good news is that depression is one of the most treatable forms of mental disorder. The use of 5-HTP to elevate serotonin levels can produce astounding results. Since I first became aware of 5-HTP's benefits in the early 1990s, I have used it to treat hundreds of depressed patients. When treatment involves a complete, well-rounded program that addresses all aspects of depression—including diet, stress management, and exercise—the "darkness visible" dissipates, and light returns again to life.

In the following pages I'll describe some key scientific studies that compared 5-HTP to other treatment methods and show you how to interpret their results. The final section of this chapter explains how to use 5-HTP as part of a broader program to correct the underlying problems that contribute to depression.

How to Read a Study

To be a smart consumer of medical information, you need to know how to read and interpret the results of scientific studies. Here's a quick lesson.

In most studies, scientists divide the patients into two groups. One group receives the active medication. The other group receives a placebo, a "dummy pill" that contains no medication. Usually neither the doctors nor the patients know which group receives the active drug and which gets the placebo. This method, called a double-blind placebo-controlled study, is a good way to test whether a treatment does any good. It eliminates bias, because neither the subjects nor their caregivers know who is receiving the "real" medication. In contrast, an open study is one in which the physicians (and sometimes the patients) know that they are receiving the active drug.

The term *controlled* means that both groups are subjected to exactly the same conditions. The only difference is that one receives an active medication and the other doesn't.

Results of a placebo-controlled study merely indicate whether treatment X produces any benefits compared to doing nothing at all. Such studies do not, however, indicate whether treatment X might actually be better than another active therapy, treatment Y. To find out which of two treatments is superior, the researchers conduct what is known as a head-to-head comparison, in which the two therapies known to produce results are pitted directly against each other. Ideally, such studies also involve a way to double-check the findings. For example, the study might include use of a placebo. Or group 1 might receive treatment X for four weeks and then switch over to treatment Y (or placebo), while group 2 receives treatment Y and then switches to treatment X (or placebo). This is known as a crossover study. If a group demonstrates positive results in the first segment of the study but not in the crossover phase, it is a sign that the first treatment might indeed offer some benefit.

Certain problems with the study can call the results into question. The size of the study is one factor. Research involving only a dozen patients might not be as valid as findings involving a hundred or more. Scientists use complicated statistical formulas to determine whether the size of the study is appropriate for the type of results they hope to produce.

Also, for results to be considered valid, the study must compare "apples to apples." That is, the groups of patients being compared should all share similar traits, such as age, the severity of their illness, the duration of treatment, and the dosage of medication they receive.

Virtually all published studies will state whether their findings are significant or not. In this context, "significant" does not necessarily mean important or that a given treatment is highly effective. The term merely indicates that, according to the strict rules of statistical analysis, the findings are not merely the result of chance or accident.

One last point: Results from a single study are not enough to base important decisions on. If findings are valid, then it should be possible for other scientists to confirm those results by conducting similarly designed studies—and coming up with similar results.

A Quick Look at Antidepressant Drugs

To understand the benefits of 5-HTP, it helps to know a little bit about the other drugs available for treating depression.

There are four basic types of antidepressants on the market (Table 2.1). The oldest drugs are known as the tricyclics. (The name refers to the fact that the molecules of the drug have a distinctive three-ring structure.) These drugs work by blocking the reuptake of the neurotransmitters serotonin and norepinephrine. Examples of the tricyclics include amitriptyline and desipramine. Generally, these drugs are effective for between 60 percent and 80 percent of the people who take them. That's about the same rate of efficacy seen in all classes of antidepressants. The tricyclics regulate mood primarily through their effects on the serotonin system. However, as I said, they also affect the other

main neurotransmitter systems. These other actions are what produce the side effects that often arise with use of the tricyclics.
About 35 to 55 percent of people taking tricyclics experience such
complications as dry mouth, nausea, increased heart rate, constipation, fatigue, and sleepiness.

Another class of antidepressants includes the monoamine oxidase (MAO) inhibitors. These drugs work in a different way from
the tricyclics. They slow down the activity of the enzyme
(monoamine oxidase) that breaks down neurotransmitter molecules as they float around in gaps between brain cells. The drugs
don't increase the levels of monoamine neurotransmitters in the
brain; they just prevent the available supply from "dissolving."
Like the tricyclics, MAO inhibitors such as phenelzine (Nardil)
and tranylcypromine (Parnate) affect all the monoamine neurotransmitters. Thus they too have a high risk of side effects. Also of
concern is the fact that certain foods contain a substance called
tyramine that affects the MAO enzyme. Such foods include beer,
aged cheese, and wine. If you eat tyramine-rich foods while taking
an MAO inhibitor, there is a risk that your blood pressure may
increase to dangerous levels, leading to cerebral hemorrhage or
abnormal heart rhythms.

Which brings us to the third class of antidepressants, the serotonin reuptake inhibitors. As the name suggests, these drugs work
by inhibiting the reabsorption of serotonin at the nerve endings in
the brain. As a result, more serotonin is available to bind to receptor sites on brain cells and transmit the serotonin signal. Drugs
such as fluoxetine (Prozac) and sertraline (Zoloft) affect only the
serotonin system, so they are classified as *selective* serotonin
reuptake inhibitors, or SSRIs. Another drug, venlafaxine (Ef-
fexor), is not selective; it inhibits reuptake of serotonin and other
monoamines as well, so it is classified as an SRI. As I've mentioned, these drugs all work in approximately the same percentage
of patients—around 70 percent. Because the selective SRIs affect
just the serotonin system, however, they are less likely to cause
the unwanted side effects seen with the tricyclics, and they do not

pose the same potentially fatal risk as the MAO inhibitors. It is this more favorable side effect profile—not a greater degree of efficacy—that accounts for the enormous popularity of Prozac and its chemical cousins during the past decade or so.

The fourth category of drug is a catchall group known as the "miscellaneous" antidepressants, because they exert a variety of effects on the neurotransmitter systems. Examples include bupropion (Wellbutrin) and trazodone (Desyrel). An antidepressant approved for use in the United States in 1996, mirtazapine (Remeron), is sometimes referred to as an NaSRI—a norepinephrine and serotonin reuptake inhibitor. No doubt we will see more variations on this theme as new drugs appear on the market in coming years, as scientists get better at targeting different drugs to different neurotransmitter systems.

Table 2.1: Categories of Prescription Antidepressant Drugs

Category	Generic Name	Brand Name(s)
Tricyclics	amitriptyline	Elavil, Endep
	clomipramine	Anafranil
	desipramine	Norpramin, Pertofrane
	doxepin	Adapin, Sinequan
	imipramine	Imavate, Presamine, Tofranil
	nortriptyline	Aventyl, Pamelor
	protriptyline	Vivactil
Monoamine oxidase inhibitors	phenelzine	Nardil
	tranylcypromine	Parnate
Serotonin reuptake inhibitors	fluoxetine	Prozac
	fluvoxamine	Luvox
	paroxetine	Paxil

	sertraline	Zoloft
	venlafaxine	Effexor
Miscellaneous	bupropion	Wellbutrin
	maprotiline	Ludiomil
	mirtazapine	Remeron
	trazodone	Desyrel

Studies on 5-HTP in Depression

Does 5-HTP relieve depression? And if so, does it do so more effectively than other treatments, including the conventional prescription antidepressants? To answer those questions, let's look first at early studies of 5-HTP.

By the late 1960s, studies on animals and humans had established the fact that low serotonin levels were involved in depression. To determine what role 5-HTP played in the serotonin-conversion process, researchers in Japan conducted an interesting study. They injected a radioactive form of 5-HTP into cats. Using special monitors, the scientists were able to discover what happened to the molecule in the cats' bodies. They discovered that the 5-HTP essentially made a beeline for the serotonin-producing cells of the brain, where it was quickly converted into serotonin.[4]

All well and good. But there were important questions yet to be addressed: Is 5-HTP safe for humans, and what effects, if any, does it produce on normal, healthy, nondepressed individuals?

To find out, researchers injected human volunteers with a dose of 200 mg of 5-HTP. Out of thirty-five test subjects, thirty-four reported immediate feelings of euphoria—that is, a sense of calmness, well-being, and mildly elevated mood. Such results suggested that 5-HTP might play an important role in helping people whose moods were depressed return to a more normal state.[5]

Some of the first clinical studies on 5-HTP for the treatment of depression began in the early 1970s in Japan under the direction of Professor Isamu Sano of the Osaka University Medical School. Sano's first study involved 107 patients with either unipolar or bipolar depression who received 5-HTP at doses ranging from 50 to 300 mg per day. Within two weeks, more than half of these patients experienced improvement in their symptoms. By the end of the four-week study, nearly three fourths of the patients— seventy-four of the one hundred seven—reported either complete relief or significant improvement. Of equal importance, the patients experienced no significant side effects.[6] Similar promising results were found in subsequent studies conducted by other researchers in Japan. Of special interest was the fact that in two of these follow-up studies, 5-HTP proved to be effective in a subgroup of patients (50 percent in one study, 35 percent in another) who had not gotten better when taking any other antidepressant drug.[7]

The most thorough of the early Japanese studies was conducted in 1978 under the direction of Teruo Nakajima, also of the Osaka University Medical School.[8] This study enrolled fifty-nine patients with depression, thirty males and twenty-nine females. Before the study, the patients rated their depression as being moderate to severe. The patients then received 5-HTP in dosages of 50 or 100 mg three times daily for at least three weeks. The antidepressant activity and clinical effectiveness of 5-HTP were then determined using a patient questionnaire. As Table 2.2 shows, the improvements among the various patients and subtypes of depression ranged from slight to marked improvement in fourteen out of seventeen patients with unipolar depression and in twelve out of twenty-one patients with bipolar depression. Comparable results were seen in the other subtypes as well. Side effects were minimal; only one patient in ten reported slight nausea.

50   100   x 3 weeks
Tid   Tid
(150mg)   (300mg)

Table 2.2: Improvement in Various Subtypes of Depression with 5-HTP Treatment

Subtype	Degree of Improvement*						
	1	2	3	4	5,6,7	8	1+2+3/ total**
First-episode depression	1	1	0	1	0	0	2/3
Unipolar depression	3	8	3	1	2	0	14/17
Bipolar depression	6	4	2	3	3	3	12/21
Mixed depression	0	1	0	1	0	0	1/2
Presenile or senile depression	3	2	0	3	1	0	5/9
Neurotic depression	0	1	2	1	0	0	3/4
Reactive depression	0	1	1	0	0	0	2/2
Schizophrenic depression	0	1	0	0	0	0	1/1
Total	13	19	8	10	6	3	40/59
% of total	22.0	32.2	13.6	16.9	10.2	5.1	67.8%

* Improvement: 1 = marked improvement; 2 = moderately improved; 3 = slightly improved; 4 = unchanged; 5,6,7 = felt worse; 8 = dropped out.

** The number of subjects that improved (improvement scores 1, 2, or 3) compared to the total number of subjects in that subtype.

Source: T. Nakajima, Y. Kudo, and Z. Kaneko, "Clinical evaluation of 5-hydroxy-L-tryptophan as an antidepressant drug," Folia Psychiatrica et Neurologica Japonica 32 (1978): 223–30.

These Japanese studies were "open" studies, which means that both doctors and patients knew what medicine was being given. And as discussed before, there is a potential for bias in analyzing the data generated by an open study.

In 1972 Herman van Praag and his colleagues at the Psychiatric University Clinic, Groningen, The Netherlands were the first to study 5-HTP in a double-blind format. In other words, neither the researchers nor the subjects knew who was getting the active product. The process began with a small preliminary study that involved ten patients hospitalized for severe, unremitting depression that was not responding to other forms of treatment.[9] Half of the subjects received 5-HTP at dosages ranging from 200 to 3,000 mg daily, while the other half received a placebo.

The results were encouraging. Three out of the five people taking 5-HTP experienced significant improvement within two weeks, while all of the patients in the placebo group got worse during the three-week study. Of particular importance was the fact that people with such severe depression—remember, they were hospitalized—usually do not experience such a quick response to standard antidepressant drugs. And when the drugs do work, positive results usually appear some time after two weeks; improvement after four to six weeks is more typical. From this preliminary study, van Praag decided that 5-HTP was worth a closer look, and since then he and his colleagues have conducted a number of clinical studies on 5-HTP and other treatments for depression.

Are Some People More Likely to Respond to 5-HTP?

Back in 1972, 5-HTP was in pretty scarce supply and was prohibitively expensive. That caused Dr. van Praag to wonder: Could there be a test that would identify which depressed people would be more likely to get better while taking the substance? Identifying such people—known as "responders"—ahead of time would be a big plus. "Nonresponders" wouldn't waste time and money taking a product that wouldn't do them any good. More important, responders could be identified and would get the relief from depression they so desperately needed.

Indeed, van Praag developed just such a test.[10] Patients undergo a procedure known as a spinal tap, during which a sample of fluid is drawn from the spinal cord and studied in a lab. The researchers measure the level of 5-HIAA (a chemical that is left over when the body breaks down molecules of serotonin). Then the patient takes a drug known as probenecid for the next three days. This drug prevents the 5-HIAA from passing out of the spinal fluid and into the bloodstream. A repeat spinal tap is performed on the fourth day. Because the 5-HIAA has been "trapped" in the fluid, the levels of this substance indicate how much serotonin has been produced by the body during the time of the study.

From the results of the probenecid test, Dr. van Praag and his colleagues discovered that the average level of 5-HIAA was significantly lower in depressed individuals compared to the levels in normal, healthy controls. Low levels of the serotonin breakdown product, in turn, were a sign that low levels of serotonin were being manufactured by the brain. Thus, 5-HIAA could serve as a biological marker for depression that resulted from low serotonin. Also important was that the researchers confirmed their theory that antidepressant therapy with 5-HTP was much more effective in patients who had low 5-HIAA levels, as measured by the probenecid test.[11]

Most people do not relish the thought of undergoing not one but *two* spinal taps and taking probenecid for three days merely to find out if they might be candidates for treatment with 5-HTP. Fortunately, you don't need to put yourself through such an ordeal. Because 5-HTP is safe and inexpensive, try taking it for a few weeks following the recommendations at the end of this chapter. If after two weeks you don't notice a response, then it may be that 5-HTP is not right for you.

For Fast Relief

As I reviewed the many studies on 5-HTP in preparation for writing this book, I was continually amazed by one consistent finding: the speed with which depressed people respond to treatment with 5-HTP. For example, in a landmark 1991 study, Walter Pöldinger and colleagues saw results within three to five days in patients taking 5-HTP, compared to four to seven days in patients taking an SSRI.[12] The Nakajima study cited earlier is another good example. Of the forty patients who responded to 5-HTP, thirty-two—80 percent of them—did so within the first two weeks of therapy (Table 2.3). In contrast, in most studies with conventional antidepressant drugs, the benefits usually are not apparent until after two to four weeks of treatment. If you review the scientific literature, you will see that most studies on antidepressants last six or eight weeks or more. That's because researchers know it takes that much time for these medications to affect brain chemistry in a significant and positive manner. Most of the 5-HTP studies, however, took less than six weeks to produce results. (This is not because the scientists were in a hurry. It is simply a reflection of the fact that statistically significant results are seen more rapidly with 5-HTP.) Even so, the longer people take 5-HTP, the better the results usually are, and some of my patients find they need to stay on 5-HTP for at least two months before they start seeing significant benefits.

Table 2.3: Elapsed Time to Improvement with 5-HTP Therapy

Degree of Improvement	Number of Patients					
	Day 1	Day 2	Day 3	Day 4-7	Day 8-14	Day 15
Marked	1	3	2	5	2	0
Moderate	0	1	13	1	4	0

| Slight | 0 | 2 | 2 | 2 | 1 | 1 |
| Total | 1 | 6 | 17 | 8 | 7 | 1 |

Source: T. Nakajima, Y. Kudo, and Z. Kaneko, "Clinical evaluation of 5-hydroxy-L-tryptophan as an antidepressant drug," Folia Psychiatrica et Neurologica Japonica 32 (1978): 223–30.

5-HTP vs. L-Tryptophan: A Double-Blind Study

In 1984 researchers at Albert Einstein College of Medicine, led by Dr. van Praag, conducted a head-to-head, double-blind study comparing the antidepressant effects of L-tryptophan and 5-HTP.[13] In Dr. van Praag's study, forty-five subjects with depression were given either L-tryptophan (5 g/day), 5-HTP (200 mg/day), or a placebo. The groups were matched according to age, sex, and severity of depression. Results were measured by asking the patients to fill out a questionnaire known as the Hamilton Rating Scale for Depression (HRSD), a widely used assessment tool in clinical research on depression.

The score for the HRSD is determined by having the test subjects rate the severity of their symptoms on a scale of 0 (not present) to 4 (very severe). Symptoms assessed by the HRSD include feelings of guilt, anxiety, insomnia, and bodily complaints such as gastrointestinal symptoms, headaches, muscle aches, heart palpitations, and so on. The researchers add the numbers and assess the severity of depression according to a scale. The subjects complete the HRSD questionnaire at the beginning and at the end of the study (and often at one or more intervals in between). Any changes noted in the scores are then subjected to statistical analysis to determine whether the results are significant.

Here are the beginning and end HRSD scores of the three groups from the van Praag study. Remember, the higher the number, the more severe the symptoms of depression.

	5-HTP	L-Tryptophan	Placebo
Beginning of the study	26	25	23
End of the study (30 days)	9	15	19

As you can see, the patients in all three groups started the study with pretty severe depression scores. But after a month of treatment, the scores for the 5-HTP group fell dramatically. The scores among the L-tryptophan group also fell, but not nearly as far. In contrast, the placebo group's scores barely moved.

Such findings provide strong evidence that treatment with 5-HTP is superior to L-tryptophan and placebo in the treatment of depression, as measured by a drop in the HRSD score. As we have seen, the reasons for this may be that 5-HTP crosses the blood-brain barrier more easily, and that doses of L-tryptophan increase the conversion of tryptophan into kynurenine (and thus prevent its conversion to serotonin).

5-HTP vs. Antidepressant Drugs

Results of dozens of scientific studies have convinced me that 5-HTP is far superior to all types of prescription antidepressant drugs—even the newer ones. Here's a quick recap of the evidence.

5-HTP VS. TRICYCLIC ANTIDEPRESSANTS

5-HTP was compared to a tricyclic antidepressant drug, imipramine, in a head-to-head comparative study conducted at the Psychiatric University Hospital in Zurich, Switzerland.[14] The investigators concluded that there was no significant difference in efficacy between 5-HTP and imipramine. 5-HTP, however, caused fewer and less severe side effects.

Dr. van Praag and his colleagues also wanted to see if 5-HTP had any advantage over the tricyclics. In their head-to-head comparison, they found that 5-HTP at daily doses of 200 mg was just as effective as the tricyclic clomipramine and that 5-HTP did not cause troublesome side effects. Intriguingly, these investigators also found that a combination of 5-HTP plus clomipramine produced better results than either compound alone.[15]

Other researchers achieved similar results by combining 5-HTP with other medications.[16] For example, in a study conducted at a major university in Spain, 5-HTP combined with an MAO inhibitor demonstrated significant advantages compared to just the MAO inhibitor alone. These results are summarized in Table 2.4.[17]

Table 2.4: Change in Hamilton Rating Scale for Depression

	5-HTP + MAO	MAO + Placebo
Initial measurement	28.67	26.33
After 8 days	16.67	19.23
After 15 days	11.77	16.03

As a naturopathic physician, I read these findings with a growing sense of excitement. The study suggested that the benefits of 5-HTP could be boosted by using the substance along with other compounds that affect the MAO enzyme. An herbal product, *Ginkgo biloba* extract, is known to do just that. I'll have more to say about this combination and others in Chapter 7.

WARNING

It is possible for serotonin levels to get too high. The result is a condition known as *serotonin syndrome,* which is characterized by confusion, fever, shivering, sweating, diarrhea, and muscle spasms. In very rare cases, serotonin syndrome can be fatal. Some reports suggest that serotonin precursors such as L-tryptophan and 5-HTP may increase the risk of serotonin syndrome.[18]

If you are taking a prescription MAO inhibitor, *do not* take 5-HTP until you consult with your doctor. The combination of higher serotonin levels and reduced breakdown of serotonin by MAO enzymes can raise serotonin too much. If you stop taking the MAO inhibitor, allow at least four weeks to elapse before starting treatment with 5-HTP, to make sure that all of the drug has had time wash out of your body.

5-HTP vs. Serotonin Reuptake Inhibitors

After the early research in the 1970s, during the 1980s 5-HTP was increasingly being regarded as a potentially valuable antidepressant that had a low incidence of side effects. A 1987 review article on 5-HTP in depression written by professors of psychology from the University of Utah and the University of California highlighted the need for well-designed double-blind, head-to-head studies of 5-HTP versus standard antidepressant drugs, especially those new kids on the block: the SSRIs, such as Prozac.[19]

In response, in 1991, researchers in Switzerland, led by Dr. Pöldinger, conducted a double-blind study comparing 5-HTP to an SSRI called fluvoxamine (Luvox).[20] In Europe, fluvoxamine is widely used as an antidepressant. Its efficacy is equal to, or perhaps better than, other SSRIs, including Prozac. In the United States, fluvoxamine is used primarily in the treatment of obsessive-compulsive disorder (OCD). OCD, an anxiety disorder that affects an estimated five million Americans, is characterized by obsessions (unwanted, recurrent, and disturbing thoughts) and compulsions (repetitive, ritualized behaviors that the person with OCD feels driven to perform). Among the more well-known manifestations of OCD are constant hand-washing and the urge to go back and check things repeatedly, such as whether the door is locked or whether the stove is turned off.

In the Swiss study, subjects received either 5-HTP (100 mg) or fluvoxamine (50 mg) three times daily for six weeks. The patients then rated their depression using such instruments as the Hamilton scale, the Self-Assessment Depression Scale (SADS), and a physician's assessment questionnaire called the Clinical Global Impression, or CGI. Let's look first at the results with the Hamilton scale.

The patients' scores on the HRSD were assessed at the beginning of the study to establish what scientists call the baseline levels. The survey was taken again at the two-, four-, and six-week marks. At the beginning, the average HRSD score for the group of patients who would be treated with 5-HTP was 27.1; among the fluvoxamine group the average score was 25.8. Both groups experienced significant improvement in their symptoms. At the end of six weeks the final average Hamilton score for the two groups were virtually identical: 10.6 for the 5-HTP group and 10.7 for the fluvoxamine group. (Remember, a drop in score means an improvement in mood.) However, because the 5-HTP group started at a higher level, their overall degree of improvement was better (a decrease of 60.7 percent compared to 56.1 percent for the fluvoxamine group). What's more, 5-HTP worked more quickly than fluvoxamine and produced a response in a higher percentage of patients. After just two weeks, the overall drop in HRSD scores was 23 percent, compared to just under 19 percent among the fluvoxamine group.

The patients were also evaluated using other types of surveys. According to the patient evaluations, in which the study subjects rated their own status, fluvoxamine came up shining. Only ten out of thirty-four patients taking 5-HTP indicated that their depression had improved by more than 75 percent. However, a larger group among the fluvoxamine group—thirteen out of twenty-nine—reported improvement of more than 75 percent. But when the physicians rated the patients' progress according to the CGI scale, they noted no difference between the two groups in the percentage of those who experienced dramatic improvement. Furthermore, according to the physicians' rating, only two out of thirty-four subjects in the 5-HTP group (about 6 percent) failed to gain benefit, while five out of twenty-nine patients on fluvoxamine (about 16 percent) failed to improve. Taking all of these measurements as a whole, the conclusion is that, while both treatments are effective, 5-HTP has the edge.

The advantages of 5-HTP over fluvoxamine are even more dramatic if we study the effects on treatment on specific symptoms of depression, as measured by the Hamilton scale: depressed mood, anxiety, physical symptoms, and insomnia. These results are summarized in Table 2.5.

Table 2.5: Improvement in Specific Depression Symptoms

Symptom	5-HTP	Fluvoxamine
Depressed mood	67.5%	61.8%
Anxiety	58.2%	48.3%
Physical symptoms	47.6%	37.8%
Insomnia	61.7%	55.9%

Source: W. Pöldinger, B. Calanchini, W. Schwartz, "A functional-dimensional approach to depression: Serotonin deficiency as a target syndrome in a comparison of 5-HTP and fluvoxamine," *Psychopathology* 24 (1991): 53–81.

Let's now look at the data from the patients' self-assessment depression scale. SADS is a questionnaire, filled out by the patient, that rates twenty symptoms of depression and weights them according to the frequency of their occurrence. According to the SADS evaluation, 5-HTP reduced depression symptoms by 53.3 percent compared to 47.6 percent for the fluvoxamine group. The SADS scale states that anything over a 50 percent drop reflects an excellent result. By this measure, which reflects how the patients themselves subjectively respond to treatment, 5-HTP was superior.

Efficacy is one concern; safety (that is, the extent of side effects) is another. In the study, the number of patients experiencing side effects was, practically speaking, the same: fifteen (38.9 percent) among the 5-HTP group reported problems, compared to eighteen (54.5 percent) of the fluvoxamine group. The most common side effects reported among the 5-HTP group were nausea, heartburn, and gastrointestinal problems (flatulence, feelings of fullness, and rumbling sensations). Patients reported that these problems were very mild or mild. In contrast, most of the side effects experienced in the fluvoxamine group were rated as being of moderate to severe intensity.

Another way to measure the success of a treatment is by the number of patients who drop out of a study. The only subject to drop out of the 5-HTP group did so after thirty-five days (five weeks), while four subjects in the fluvoxamine group dropped out after only two weeks. Such results suggest that 5-HTP may be better tolerated for longer periods than treatment with an SSRI.

5-HTP in the Long Term

One of the big problems with depression is that it can be a lifelong, recurrent illness. Some patients with severe depression suffer from frequent bouts of depression. Their moods will lift, only to plunge again into darkness a few months later. Such patients typically require constant use of treatment, including medications and counseling. Even with this support, relapses are still a problem. This raises a question: Is 5-HTP valuable for the long-term treatment of depression as a way of preventing relapse?

To answer that question, Dr. van Praag conducted a two-year double-blind study in twenty patients with long-standing unipolar or bipolar depression.[21] Group A received 5-HTP at a dosage of 200 mg per day for one year followed by a one-year period on a placebo. Group B took the placebo for the first phase of the study and 5-HTP for the second. During the treatment phases, there were a total of seven relapses in the two groups. In startling contrast, during the placebo period, the total number of relapses was 24—more than one for each patient. Dr. van Praag further demonstrated that the best results were achieved in the patients who had low serotonin levels, as determined by the probenecid test I described earlier (see box, page 59). Among these thirteen low-serotonin patients, only one experienced a relapse of depression during treatment with 5-HTP.

5-HTP in Therapy-Resistant Depression

As I have mentioned, most methods of treating depression are effective about 60 to 80 percent of the time. That means, for example, that on average perhaps three out of ten people taking Prozac will not get better. The standard approach in such cases is to try another drug. Of the 30 percent or so who do not improve on an SSRI, perhaps seven out of ten will get results by switching to an MAO inhibitor. In some patients, though, it seems that nothing will work. Patients who do not improve after repeated treatments are known as "therapy-resistant."

Fortunately, evidence is mounting that 5-HTP might work even in patients who have responded to no other method. Some studies show that, for these patients, 5-HTP might work alone or in combination with a standard antidepressant.

One of the more impressive recent studies involved ninety-nine patients whom their doctors described as suffering from therapy-resistant depression.[22] The label seemed to fit; these patients had not responded to any previous therapy including all available antidepressant drugs and electroconvulsive therapy (ECT, or electrical shock treatment). These patients then received 5-HTP at an average daily dose of 200 mg (range 50 mg to 600 mg per day). According to the authors of the study, forty-three of the ninety-nine patients experienced a complete recovery. Another eight experienced significant improvement. Thus more than 50 percent of the people who failed to get better on standard treatments saw their depression lift while taking 5-HTP.

One amazing note about these results: On average, these people had suffered from depression *for a period of nine years!* They had tried everything, and nothing had helped until they received 5-HTP. I'd also like to emphasize that one of the real benefits of treatment with 5-HTP is the marked improvement in the quality of sleep. Since these patients were able to enjoy sound, restful sleep, they were more likely to wake up in the morning feeling refreshed and energetic. I'll have much more to say about the importance of sleep and the serotonin system in Chapter 4.

I'm not the only one who was amazed by the results. The author, Dr. J. J. van Hiele, states quite clearly:

> [5-HTP] merits a place in the front of the ranks of the antidepressants instead of being used as a last resort. . . . I have never in 20 years used an agent which: (1) was effective so quickly; (2) restored the patients so completely to the persons they had been and their partners had known; [and] (3) was so entirely without side effects.

Side Effects of Antidepressant Therapy

The goal of any treatment for any medical condition is to gain the most benefit while minimizing the impact of side effects to the greatest extent possible. Doctors refer to this as the "risk-benefit ratio": The benefits of a therapy should outweigh the inconvenience (or dangers) of side effects.

It's a basic fact of medicine that any treatment strong enough to produce a desired effect in the body is also strong enough to produce unwanted effects. When it comes to treatment of depression, whether with 5-HTP or any other medication, most people find that improved mood, greater energy, and a better quality of sleep are benefits that far outweigh the potential problems associated with side effects. Still, the best treatment approach is the one that yields the greatest good while reducing the risk of adverse reactions to the lowest possible level.

The main problem with the older antidepressants—the tricyclics—is that they cause extreme dry mouth in nearly two out of three patients. Dizziness, constipation, and nausea are the other main complaints with the tricyclics.

Generally, patients find they are better able to tolerate the SSRIs, such as Prozac, than the tricyclics or the MAO inhibitors. But problems with side effects still exist with these medications. As many as 17 percent of patients taking SSRIs eventually stop taking the drug because of complaints about side effects. The main reported adverse effects of the serotonin-specific antidepressants include nausea, headaches, anxiety and nervousness, insomnia, drowsiness, diarrhea, dry mouth, sweating and tremors, and skin rashes (Table 2.6).[23]

There's another serious problem. Antidepressants, especially Prozac and other SSRIs, have a profound effect on sexuality. Specifically, many people taking these drugs complain that they have severely reduced sexual desire. Even if they feel like having sex, the drugs apparently affect the nerves and muscles associated with sexual activity. Many men taking SSRIs are unable to achieve and sustain an erection. Men and women both may be less able— or completely unable—to achieve orgasm. When Prozac originally hit the market, the sexual side effects were not widely reported; only about 1 percent or so of patients mentioned it in the original preclinical trials. But now that we've had about a decade of clinical experience with the drug, the pattern is clear. In studies where sexual side effects were thoroughly evaluated, 43 percent of people taking drugs for depression, and 34 percent of people taking Prozac, reported loss of libido or diminished sexual response.[24] Some experts believe that the rate of sex-related adverse effects with Prozac might be as high as 75 percent.[25]

More important is that loss of interest in sex is one of the more troubling symptoms of depression—it should not also be a by-product of treatment! Depression makes its victims feel a profound loss of pleasure in everyday activities. Loss of sexuality can trigger a range of associated problems: feelings of guilt or shame, withdrawal from a spouse or partner, increased isolation and loneliness, a sense of hopelessness and despair. These are some of the very issues that treatment for depression is intended to address.

Table 2.6: Side Effects of 5-HTP, Tricyclics, and SSRIs

Side Effect	% of Patients Experiencing Side Effect		
	5-HTP	Tricyclics	SSRIs
Nausea	9	15	23
Headache	5	16	20
Nervousness	2.5	11	16
Insomnia	2.5	7	17
Anxiety	2.5	9	14
Drowsiness	7	23	11
Diarrhea	2.5	4	12
Tremor	0	18	11
Dry mouth	7	64.5	12
Sweating	2.5	15	9
Dizziness	5	25.5	7
Constipation	5	25	5.5
Vision changes	0	14.5	4

Sources: G. D. Tollefson et al., "Evaluation of suicidality during pharmacologic treatment of mood and nonmood disorders," *Annals of Clinical Psychiatry* 5 (1993): 209–24; W. Pöldinger, B. Calanchini, and W. Schwartz, "A functional-dimensional approach to depression: Serotonin deficiency as a target syndrome in a comparison of 5-HTP and fluvoxamine," *Psychopathology* 24 (1991): 53–81.

Restoring Sexuality:

ROGER'S STORY

Roger felt as though he'd been hit by a triple whammy. He had just turned fifty. For this active, energetic man, being "half a century old," as he put it, had made him start thinking about his own mortality.

Then the company where he'd worked for the past seventeen years, a leading manufacturer of camera equipment, announced that it was being bought by a conglomerate. Roger had worked his way up to regional sales manager, and despite the company's assurances that "everyone's job was safe," he was deeply worried that he was about to be downsized out of a job. He wasn't sleeping well and was having real trouble concentrating at work. Three months before, his family doctor had started him on Zoloft (sertraline), an antidepressant that, like Prozac, is a serotonin reuptake inhibitor.

And lately . . . well, lately he hadn't been feeling much like "a man."

During his visit to my office, Roger didn't bring up the subject of sex until late in our conversation. He had made the appointment, he said, because he wanted to talk about the nutritional supplements he was taking. Just as we were winding up, though, he asked whether I thought any of the supplements in his regimen would help bring back some zest to his love life.

I probed a little further. Gradually he told the whole story: The Zoloft had helped with the depression, no doubt about it. "The drug really takes care of the lows," he said. "But it also pretty much wipes out the highs. Everything becomes kind of, I don't know, flat." He supposed he could deal with that, he said. But over the past couple of months his interest in sex—usually pretty high, he confessed—had dwindled. "Even when the spirit is willing," he said, "the flesh is kinda weak."

Like many men, Roger felt that, to a significant degree, his identity as a man was tied up with his ability to function sexually. Rightly or wrongly, sex is often at the center of a man's self-image. For Roger, loss of sexual appetite and function robbed him of his self-esteem and made him feel embarrassed and ashamed.

I had seen this pattern before. Although sexual problems can be symptoms of the debilitating illness we call depression, they can also arise as side effects of treatment with prescription antidepressants. I suggested that Roger talk to his family doctor about discontinuing the Zoloft. The doctor agreed and had him cut the daily dose in half for two weeks, then take a dose only every other day for another two weeks, then stop altogether. In the meantime I started Roger on a regimen of 5-HTP, 100 mg a day at bedtime.

Roger came to see me again not long ago. This time he didn't wait till the end of our session to talk about his sex life. "It's nice to have those highs back again," he said with a smile.

The Long View

We do not yet have long-term studies on the use of SSRIs in people. In a sense, patients taking these drugs over the course of years are like guinea pigs; researchers are waiting to see if using an SSRI for a long time poses special risk. A recent study in animals suggests there may be cause to worry. Dr. Lorne Brandes of the Manitoba Institute of Cell Biology in Winnipeg found that animals receiving doses of Prozac and other antidepressants at levels comparable to those given to humans had significantly greater growth of cancerous tumors.[26] The rate of tumor growth was also greater than it was in a control group of animals that did not receive Prozac. Much more research needs to be done before we can conclude that antidepressants cause cancer, but such findings raise troubling concerns about the long-term safety of these medications.

As you've seen from the previous discussion, 5-HTP poses a

much lower risk of side effects than other available standard antidepressants. Let's address the sexual issue first: 5-HTP has not been associated with decreased sexual drive and performance. For example, a study conducted at the University of Munich demonstrated no adverse effects on sexual function when 5-HTP was given to healthy volunteers.[27] In fact, many of my patients have reported that their sexual energy and interest have been enhanced while taking 5-HTP. But the scientific evidence for this is indirect; it comes from research on L-tryptophan. In these case reports, both normal and depressed people (men and women) taking L-tryptophan reported increased libido (sexual drive).[28] From my experience, though, I believe that if L-tryptophan produces these positive effects, then 5-HTP will produce even better results.

As Table 2.6 shows, the most frequently reported side effect with 5-HTP is nausea. The problem of nausea is a theme of all treatments that affect the serotonin system. One reason, as you learned in Chapter 1, is that serotonin is very active in cells of the digestive system. About 30 percent of an oral dose of 5-HTP is converted to serotonin in the intestinal tract. It appears that a sudden increase in the level of this powerful neurotransmitter in this part of the body can trigger sensations that are perceived as mild nausea. Actually, the rate of nausea due to 5-HTP is lower than that experienced with other antidepressant drugs. For example, while about one in ten people taking 300 mg of 5-HTP a day might notice nausea, the rate among people taking standard doses of Prozac is about 23 percent, or one in four. Here's another surprising but important finding: In double-blind studies, the incidence of nausea among the group taking the inactive placebo—an inactive substance—is *also* around 10 percent.

Reducing the Risk of Nausea

In my practice, I find that most patients tolerate 5-HTP very well; the rate of nausea reported by my patients is considerably less than 10 percent. Those who do experience nausea report that the problem tends to disappear after a couple of weeks of treatment as the body gets used to the presence of the substance. And from my years of experience in treating patients with 5-HTP, I've learned that there are some things you can do to reduce the risk even further.

Following the right dosage schedule helps a lot. When I prescribe 5-HTP for depression, I recommend a starting dosage of 50 mg three times per day. If needed, after two weeks of use, you can try increasing the dosage to 100 mg three times per day. Taking 5-HTP with food helps reduce its absorption by the digestive system, so I usually recommend taking the dose at the beginning of a meal or about twenty minutes before.

A well-known natural method of reducing nausea is to take doses of ginger. For more information on ginger, see Chapter 7.

Lastly, if you have a sensitive stomach, it may be a good idea to take 5-HTP pills that are enteric-coated. This means that the pill has a special shell that prevents it from dissolving immediately in the stomach. The active ingredient will not be released until the pill passes into the small intestine, which does not contain 5-HTP-responsive cells.

5-HTP vs. Antidepressant Drugs: Conclusions

In terms of its effectiveness in treating depression, 5-HTP has been shown to be just as effective as the established drugs—the SSRIs, the MAO inhibitors, and the tricyclic antidepressants. The advantages of 5-HTP lie in the fact that 5-HTP is better tolerated and is associated with fewer and much milder side effects. And frankly, many people find it reassuring to use a naturally occurring, naturally derived substance like 5-HTP instead of a synthetic drug.

Enhancing 5-HTP with Catecholamine Precursors

In the early 1970s Dr. van Praag and his associates were getting very good results by treating depressed people with 5-HTP. But they noticed a disturbing pattern. In about one patient out of five who responded to 5-HTP, the benefits started to decrease after a month or so of treatment. As the 5-HTP "wore off," the black clouds of depression rolled back in.[29]

Puzzled, the researchers did some further tests. They discovered a troubling fact: In these patients, the levels of serotonin had risen and had stayed high, but the levels of other important monoamine neurotransmitters, dopamine and norepinephrine, had declined. That led the researchers to wonder whether it might be possible to adjust the levels of these neurotransmitters in the same way as serotonin—that is, by providing the body with an increased supply of the raw materials (known as "precursors") it needs to make them.

Here's another quick lesson in biochemistry. Dopamine and norepinephrine, classified as catecholamines, are closely related to each other. The body manufactures them when enzymes act on an amino acid called phenylalanine. The steps in the conversion process are as follows:

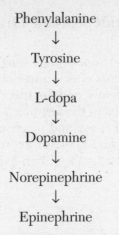

Phenylalanine
↓
Tyrosine
↓
L-dopa
↓
Dopamine
↓
Norepinephrine
↓
Epinephrine

Van Praag wondered if administering tyrosine would increase the levels of catecholamines, in the same way that giving L-tryptophan (or 5-HTP) increases the levels of serotonin. The goal was to improve the outcome for patients in whom the antidepressant benefits of 5-HTP wore off after a few weeks. As it turned out, the theory was right: Giving patients the catecholamine precursors tyrosine (more accurately, its synthesized form, known as L-tyrosine) or phenylalanine restored the effects of 5-HTP.[30]

In this study, the dosage of 5-HTP was 200 mg per day and 100 mg of L-tyrosine per kilogram (2.2 pounds) of body weight. For a 150-pound person, that means the daily dosage of L-tyrosine would be 6.8 grams per day. That is quite high, and in my experience such doses may not be necessary. Lower doses appear to be equally effective, especially if taken with a high-protein meal. Eating protein increases the rate at which tyrosine is transported across the blood-brain barrier. In contrast, as we discussed in Chapter 1, eating tryptophan-rich foods (or taking L-tryptophan supplements) can actually slow down the rate of amino acid passage into the brain.

You might wonder: If these precursors contribute to the effectiveness of treatment, do they work by themselves to relieve depression? The answer is yes. In several clinical studies that examined this question, researchers concluded that either L-tyrosine or D,L-phenylalanine used alone produced improvements in mood comparable to those seen with antidepressant drugs, but without the side effects (Table 2.7).[31] The reason appears to be that tyrosine and phenylalanine have many roles in the body. Besides being converted to dopamine and norepinephrine, they can be converted to other substances that have stimulant and mood-elevating properties. Phenylalanine (both in its D- and L-forms) increases the level of phenylethylamine (PEA), while L-tyrosine increases the levels of PEA and two other neurotransmitters, octopamine and tyramine. These compounds have stimulant and mood-elevating properties, and depressed patients have been found to have low levels of them.

Although these substances are effective on their own, my recommendation is to use L-tyrosine or D,L-phenylalanine along with 5-HTP as detailed above.

Table 2.7: Phenylalanine and Tyrosine in Depression

Substance Tested	Dose mg/day	Number Patients	Duration (days)	Results
D,L-phenylalanine	200–400	15	14	10 of 15 (66%) severely depressed patients responded
D or D,L-phenylalanine	100	23	1–13	A complete response was observed in 17 of 23 (74%) patients previously unresponsive to tricyclics and MAO inhibitors
D,L-phenylalanine	75–200	20	20	Out of 20 patients, 8 (40%) had complete remissions and another 4 (20%), marked improvement, using depression rating scales
D-phenylalanine	100–400	55	60–180	40 (73%) recovered completely after 15 days, 13 (23%) had marked improvement, 2 (4%) failed to respond
D-phenylalanine	100	60	30	83% of the phenylalanine group had complete remission and improvement compared to 73% for the imipramine group
D,L-phenylalanine	200	27	30	No significant difference between phenylalanine and imipramine groups
Tyrosine	≅6 g	9	ongoing	60–70% response rate

Sources: Data summarized from C. Gibson and A. Gelenberg, "Tyrosine for depression," *Advances in Biological Psychiatry* 10 (1983): 148–59; H. Beckman, "Phenylalanine in affective disorders," *Advances in Biological Psychiatry* 10 (1983): 137–47.

5-HTP and Decarboxylase Inhibitors

Recently some scare stories have circulated in the lay press stating that 5-HTP might be dangerous unless it is taken along with a type of drug known as a decarboxylase inhibitor. These drugs work by interfering with the activity of an enzyme that breaks down 5-HTP molecules. According to one researcher's theory, 5-HTP taken without a decarboxylase inhibitor can result in dangerous blood clots or strokes. There is also a question about whether 5-HTP would be more effective if taken along with a decarboxylase inhibitor.

However, scientific research does not bear out these notions. A study by Zmilacher and colleagues found no evidence that taking a decarboxylase inhibitor called benserazide along with 5-HTP offers any advantage.[32] In fact, the opposite appears to be true: In a number of studies, 5-HTP alone was found to be a more effective antidepressant than 5-HTP plus the enzyme inhibitor. What's more, 5-HTP alone has a better safety record than the combination. In the Zmilacher study, five out of thirteen patients taking 5-HTP alone reported a total of nine different side effects, primarily nausea and diarrhea. In contrast, six of thirteen patients taking the combination of 5-HTP + benserazide reported a total of nineteen different side effects, including acute anxiety, low-grade mania, insomnia, tension, anxiety, blurred vision, fatigue, and dizziness. None of the 5-HTP patients reported such neurological symptoms. As I interpret these findings, adding decarboxylase inhibitors to a 5-HTP regimen is unnecessary.

A More Comprehensive View of Treatment for Depression

Depression is a multifactorial illness. In other words, many factors—emotional as well as physical—contribute to its onset, its severity, and its impact on a person's life. The best and most effective way of treating depression is to see the problem in its full context and address all of the contributing factors. Effective as it is, 5-HTP is just one element in an overall treatment plan. A complete program for relieving and preventing depression is built on what I call the Four Cornerstones of Health:

- Physiology
- Attitude
- Exercise
- Nutrition

Depression results from problems affecting both the body and the mind. Physiological aspects of depression involve not just hormonal, nutritional, and chemical factors but such concerns as breathing patterns, posture, and muscle tension as well. In addition, depression can stem from, or be made worse by, our attitude, our internal focus. The types of images that we hold up to the mind's eye and the content of the internal messages we send to ourselves (self-talk) can dampen our mood and crush our spirit.

Clearly, these two levels are intertwined. Self-talk that is loaded with negative messages—"I'm a failure; no one loves me; life is not worth living"—will have a profound impact on the way our bodies function. By the same token, if our hearts do not beat strongly, our lungs do not take in an adequate supply of life-giving oxygen, and our stomachs are filled with nonnutritious foods that cannot supply necessary energy to our muscles and organs, then our brains cannot work at full capacity. It's a vicious cycle—but a cycle that can be broken.

Overcoming depression means developing positive internal images while correcting physiological problems. I view 5-HTP as a powerful tool in the treatment of depression because it addresses both the physiological and the emotional aspects of the disorder: 5-HTP is a natural way to use the body's own processes to correct an imbalance in brain chemistry, which in turn helps promote a positive attitude. By restoring a brighter outlook on life, 5-HTP provides the motivation and energy needed to take the other steps necessary to achieving a higher level of happiness.

Physiology

Before you begin any treatment for depression, including treatment with 5-HTP, it's important that you undergo a thorough medical checkup. The list of physical (organic) illnesses that can produce depression as a symptom is quite long (Table 2.8). For example, an underactive thyroid gland can have a profound impact on mood. Correcting the thyroid problem can alleviate the depression. Similarly, many drugs—including prescription and nonprescription medications, alcohol, and illicit drugs—can affect brain chemistry in such a way as to trigger depression. Knowing whether an underlying organic cause of depression is present is essential for effective treatment.

Table 2.8: Organic Causes of Depression

Cancer
Chronic inflammation
Chronic pain
Diabetes
Drugs
   Alcohol
   Anti-inflammatory agents
   Antihistamines
   Antihypertensives

Birth control pills
Cocaine
Corticosteroids
Marijuana
Tranquilizers and sedatives
Exposure to heavy metals (such as lead)
Food allergies
Heart disease
Hypoglycemia
Hypothyroidism
Liver disease
Lung disease
Multiple sclerosis
Nutritional deficiencies
Premenstrual syndrome
Rheumatoid arthritis
Sleep disturbances
Stress/low adrenal function

For a more in-depth discussion about depression arising from organic disorders or from the use of drugs and medications, you might want to read my books *Natural Alternatives to Prozac* (Morrow, 1996), *Natural Alternatives to Over-the-Counter and Prescription Drugs* (Morrow, 1994), and the *Encyclopedia of Natural Medicine* (Prima, 1998). If you are taking any medication, ask your doctor or pharmacist if the drug might cause depression as a side effect. For most health conditions, there are alternative natural medicines available that may produce better results with a lower risk of side effects than you will experience with drugs.

Attitude

Why are so many Americans depressed? I believe one of the main contributing problems is that these people feel that they personally lack the ability to control their world and how they respond to challenges. In other words, depression arises from a sense of helplessness. In a sense, growth into adulthood and maturity is, by definition, a process of gaining personal control over everything from our bodies and emotions to our careers and relationships. A person who feels that "nothing I do matters" or that "I have no purpose in life" is very vulnerable to depression.

LEARNED HELPLESSNESS

For some people, helplessness is a habit. Evidence that helplessness can be learned—and more important, that it can be *un*-learned—comes from laboratory research on animals. The pioneer in this field is Martin Seligman, Ph.D. During the 1960s Dr. Seligman conducted experiments in which caged rats were subjected to electric shocks. Some of the cages had switches that allowed the rats to turn off the shocks. In cages without the switches, the rats soon learned that there was nothing they could do to prevent the inevitable pain. These rats developed the rodent equivalent of human depression: They became lethargic, withdrawn, and unresponsive. Studies found that these depressed rats had the same types of chemical imbalances seen in their human counterparts. In contrast, the rats who had control over their environment did not become depressed.

This animal model became the main method for testing the effects of new antidepressant drugs. Rats trained to be helpless were given the test substances. If the drug worked, the animals would start exerting control over their environment again. Tests on their brains and body fluids indicated that the drugs had restored the proper balance of monoamine neurotransmitters.

Of equal significance: The animals could also learn how to regain control—and their brain chemistry would return to normal—using nondrug methods. For example, the scientists taught them to jump over the barrier or press a lever that ended the pain. Once rats learned these ways of controlling their environment, their serotonin levels rose as much as if they had been given antidepressant drugs.

Scientists soon applied these lab results to human beings. Dr. Seligman found that one of the key things that determines how people react to uncontrollable events is what he called their explanatory style—the way they explain the events to themselves. Depending on a person's style, the same event might be interpreted as good or bad. Take getting fired from a job, for example. Some people might react by feeling that the world had just caved in, that they were failures, that nothing ever went right for them. Others might react by seeing an opportunity to explore a new career, to relocate to a more desirable part of the world, or to finally get out from under the thumb of a tyrannical boss. The circumstances are the same, but the reactions are very different.

Not surprisingly, research shows that people who have a strong sense of learned helplessness are more likely to become extremely depressed when things go wrong in their lives. In contrast, people who are optimistic have a strong immunity to helplessness and depression. Optimistic individuals also have a lower risk of other serious and chronic illnesses.[33]

Just as it is possible to learn helplessness, it is possible to learn optimism. One way to start is to read some books on the subject. Dr. Seligman himself has written two important works, *Learned Optimism* (Knopf, 1991) and *What You Can Change and What You Can't* (Knopf, 1993). Your local library or bookseller can help you find other titles.

In addition, I recommend listening to motivational and/or relaxation tapes on a regular basis, especially if you are in your car a lot. The inspirational messages they contain provide a solid foundation for a positive attitude—a prime ingredient in a complete program for fighting depression.

SELF-TALK

There's a story about a psychiatrist who was treating a patient for depression. One day after a session the doctor was typing up her notes. "Patient talks to himself," she wrote. "This is not a problem. Patient does not listen to himself. *This* is the problem."

We all talk to ourselves. A constant dialogue churns in our heads. As the psychiatrist in the little story understood, this trait is a normal and healthy part of being human.

But sometimes the dialogue we have with ourselves can become toxic. Imagine a parent who constantly criticizes a child: "You never do anything right! You're clumsy and stupid! You're a loser! You'll never amount to anything!" Indeed, most children reared in such an environment will probably grow up to be insecure, unsuccessful, depressed individuals.

Negative self-talk works the same way. If we constantly feed ourselves harmful messages, we risk "poisoning the well" of our subconscious minds. One all-too-common result: depression.

Just as you can develop muscles by exercising them, it is possible to train yourself to conduct a positive inner dialogue and develop healthier attitudes. Basically the steps are to set attainable goals, pay attention to self-talk, and to recite affirmative statements that have meaning for you.

THE IMPORTANCE OF COUNSELING

Very often when I treat patients for depression, I recommend that they also see a counselor (psychotherapist). The main strategy these professionals use to help people overcome depression is known as cognitive therapy. *Cognitions* are your whole system of thoughts, beliefs, mental images, and feelings. In the treatment of moderate depression, cognitive therapy can be as effective as the use of antidepressant drugs, and there is a lower risk of relapse—the return of depression—with cognitive therapy. One reason is that cognitive therapy teaches people practical skills they can use to combat depression anytime, anywhere, every day for the rest of their lives.[34]

Mental health specialists trained in cognitive therapy seek to change the way the depressed person consciously thinks about failure, defeat, loss, and helplessness. To do so, they employ five basic tactics that help patients to:

- Recognize the negative automatic thoughts that flit through consciousness at the times when they feel the worst
- Dispute the negative thoughts by focusing on contrary evidence
- Learn a different explanation to dispute the negative automatic thoughts[35]
- Avoid rumination (the constant churning of a thought in one's mind) by helping the patients better control their thoughts
- Question depression-causing negative thoughts and beliefs, and replace them with empowering positive thoughts and beliefs

Cognitive therapy avoids the long, drawn-out (and expensive) process of psychoanalysis. It is a practical, solution-oriented psychotherapy that teaches skills a person can apply to improve the quality of life. If your thought processes are in need of a little rewiring, consider consulting a mental health professional who specializes in cognitive therapy.

Exercise

Regular exercise may be the most powerful natural antidepressant available. There is no getting around it: Our bodies and our minds require physical exercise to function properly. The physical benefits of exercise are well documented and include reduced risk for heart disease, obesity, and osteoporosis. Less generally known, but equally well documented, are the impressive mood-elevating effects of exercise. Studies show that increased participation in exercise, sports, and other physical activities strongly reduces symptoms of anxiety (restlessness, tension, etc.), depression (feelings that life is not worthwhile, low spirits, etc.), and malaise (run-down feeling, insomnia, etc.).[36] Furthermore, people who participate in regular exercise have higher self-esteem. They simply feel better and are much happier compared to people who do not exercise.

To a very large degree, the mood-elevating effects of exercise are due to a subsequent increase in the level of endorphins circulating in the body. We discussed this topic briefly in the previous chapter. A recent study found that men who jogged had less depression and less stress in their lives compared to nonjogging sedentary men of the same age. The improved mood among the runners correlated with the fact that they had lower levels of stress-related hormones and higher levels of beta-endorphins.[37] As the authors state, the outcome of the study "reaffirms that depression is very sensitive to exercise and helps firm up a biochemical link between physical activity and depression."

There have been at least a hundred clinical studies where an exercise program has been used in the treatment of depression. Overall, such studies confirm that exercise alone can be as effective as antidepressant drugs—and exercise does not cause side effects. (Of course, there is a risk of physical injury during exercise, especially if you push yourself too hard. And people with a physical condition such as heart disease should exercise caution, if you'll excuse the pun. Before undertaking any new exercise program, check with your doctor.)

Unfortunately, depression causes such symptoms as lethargy, withdrawal from activity, and a general "slowing down." Thus it is often extremely difficult for depressed people to motivate themselves to exercise, even though doing so would go a long way toward relieving their suffering.

Again, 5-HTP comes to the rescue! Treatment with this natural product elevates mood, improves sleep quality, and boosts energy levels. Using 5-HTP won't build up your biceps or give you washboard abs, but often it can provide the extra push you need to get the ball rolling and resume physical activities—for health and enjoyment.

Talk to your health care provider before beginning an exercise program. As a rule, the best all-around exercises are strength training (weight lifting) or aerobic activities such as walking briskly, jogging, bicycling, cross-country skiing, swimming, aerobic dance, and racquet sports. The basic strategy is to do an exercise that raises your heart rate to an appropriate level. For more information, see the recommendations in Chapter 3, page 136–137.

Nutrition

Good, balanced nutrition is essential for health. Imbalances in many types of nutrients can contribute to problems maintaining elevated mood.

One of the most basic issues is that, to function optimally, the brain requires a constant supply of sugars, which it extracts from the rich network of blood vessels that supply it. Consequently, low blood sugar (hypoglycemia) must be avoided. In addition to depression, symptoms of severe hypoglycemia include anxiety, irritability, fatigue, headache, blurred vision, excessive sweating, mental confusion, incoherent speech, bizarre behavior, and convulsions. Unfortunately, even though the association between hypoglycemia and depression has been well documented, few physicians consider low blood sugar as a possible factor when working up patients for depression.[38]

The following questionnaire is a useful method of identifying people at risk of hypoglycemia.

Hypoglycemia Questionnaire

No = 0   Mild = 1   Moderate = 2   Severe = 3

Crave sweets	0	1	2	3
Irritable if a meal is missed	0	1	2	3
Feel tired or weak if a meal is missed	0	1	2	3
Dizziness when standing suddenly	0	1	2	3
Frequent headaches	0	1	2	3
Poor memory (forgetful) or concentration	0	1	2	3
Feel tired an hour or so after eating	0	1	2	3
Heart palpitations	0	1	2	3
Feel shaky at times	0	1	2	3
Afternoon fatigue	0	1	2	3
Vision blurs on occasion	0	1	2	3
Depression or mood swings	0	1	2	3
Overweight	0	1	2	3
Frequently anxious or nervous	0	1	2	3
Subtotal				TOTAL:

Instructions: Circle the number that most accurately indicates the severity of each symptom. Add the scores and place the total at the bottom of each column, then add the numbers across to get your total score.

Scoring:

> 5 or less = Hypoglycemia is not likely to be a factor in depression
> 6–15 = Hypoglycemia is somewhat likely
> 16 or more = Hypoglycemia is extremely likely

If you scored 6 or higher on the hypoglycemia questionnaire, you should consider taking steps to regulate your blood sugar levels.

In most cases, all you may need to do is pay a little more attention to your diet.

CARBOHYDRATES AND DEPRESSION

Carbohydrates are the main source of sugars in the diet. In the American diet, the largest source of carbohydrates are the simple sugars, which come from such foods as white sugar, white bread, pastries, and processed breakfast cereals. Other sources are the sweeteners added to many foods, such as sucrose, glucose, maltose, lactose, and fructose (-*ose* is a chemical ending indicating sugar). The body breaks these sugars down very quickly. But these sugars contain none of the other nutrients that your body needs. They add calories but no nutrition. A healthy diet is one that restricts intake of simple sugars to the lowest possible levels.

In contrast, complex carbohydrates, or starches, are much better for you. The body breaks down complex carbohydrates more gradually, which leads to better blood sugar control. Vegetables, legumes (peas and beans), and whole grains are excellent sources of complex carbohydrates. Increasing your intake of these foods can help you raise blood sugar to an appropriate level while providing you with many other important vitamins and minerals.

Low serotonin levels are associated with powerful cravings for carbohydrates. Taking 5-HTP raises serotonin levels and helps bring these cravings under control. I'll say more about this in Chapter 3.

NUTRITION AND THE BRAIN

Besides glucose, your brain needs a constant supply of oxygen and other nutrients. Some of these nutrients are needed to help the passage of signals between nerve cells. Others, such as compounds produced from amino acids, are involved in the manufacture of neurotransmitters and other crucial chemicals.

A lack of virtually any vitamin or mineral can impair mental function to a greater or lesser degree, leading to depression, anxiety, and other mental problems. According to Melvin Werbach, M.D., a faculty member at the UCLA School of Medicine and author of *Nutritional Influences on Mental Illness: A Sourcebook of Clinical Research,* "It is clear that nutrition can powerfully influence cognition, emotion, and behavior. It is also clear that the effects of classical nutritional deficiency diseases upon mental function constitute only a small part of a rapidly expanding list of interfaces between nutrition and the mind."[39]

Dr. Werbach reports that anywhere between 31 and 68 percent of depressed people have some kind of nutritional deficiency. The most common nutritional problems associated with depression are deficiencies of folic acid, vitamin B_{12}, and vitamin B_6. It should not surprise you to learn that these substances are critically important if your body is to manufacture adequate supplies of serotonin and other neurotransmitters.

Recommendations for a Complete, Natural Approach to Relieving Depression

If you are suffering from depression, see a qualified health professional to get checked for any underlying disease or other medical condition. It is necessary to rule out such problems as low thyroid activity or diabetes.

Assuming no underlying organic illness is present, the next steps are to address the issues of mental attitude, lifestyle, and nutrition.

Develop a positive, optimistic mental attitude. Set realistic goals, and reward yourself for attaining them. Use positive self-talk and affirmations and ask yourself empowering questions. Find ways to interject humor and laughter in your life. Consider seeking the help of a mental health professional who can teach you new skills for changing the negative images and thoughts that interfere with happiness. Perform mental relaxation and stress reduction exercises such as those described in Chapter 4.

Make whatever changes you need in your lifestyle. Do not use tobacco in any form; if necessary, seek help to quit smoking. If you drink alcohol, do so only in moderation. Avoid caffeine and other stimulants. Get regular exercise.

Take a close look at your diet and see what improvements you can make. Eliminate refined sugars; instead choose whole fresh fruits and vegetables and other sources of complex carbohydrates. If you choose not to eat meat, make sure your diet contains an adequate supply of proteins, especially those that provide the essential amino acids. If you elect to supplement your diet, follow the guidelines outlined in Chapter 7.

Taking 5-HTP is a safe, effective way to increase your brain's natural antidepressants, the monoamine neurotransmitters. My standard recommendation for adults is to start by taking doses of 50 mg three times per day.

If needed, after two weeks, increase the dosage of 5-HTP to 100 mg three times per day. By gradually increasing the dosage in this way, you minimize the risk of mild nausea, which is a common reaction to higher serotonin levels. It also helps to take your dose of 5-HTP along with your meal. Do not take the full daily dose (150–300 mg) all at once. Doing so can raise the risk of nausea and will not provide additional benefits, since higher doses do not necessarily pass through the blood-brain barrier more quickly. (For more information on nausea, see the box on page 76.)

If you are not satisfied with the results, you can consider increasing the dosage. The maximum dose I would recommend for depression is 150 mg of 5-HTP four times daily (total daily dose 600 mg) for two weeks. If this dosage works for you, great. If not, then you may want to consider adding an herbal medicine. Typically, for people over the age of fifty, I recommend *Ginkgo biloba* extract. If the patient is under the age of fifty, I usually suggest St.-John's-wort extract. Both of these wonderful herbal medicines are available in combination with 5-HTP and are described more fully in Chapter 7.

If you notice that the benefits of 5-HTP seem to wear off after one month, I recommend that you supplement the treatment by taking 500 mg of L-tyrosine or 100 mg of D,L-phenylalanine three times daily.

Cautions

In most cases, 5-HTP produces results within two weeks, but in some cases people may need to take it for eight weeks before their depression lifts. Do not take 5-HTP if you are taking a prescription antidepressant, especially an MAO inhibitor, without first talking to the prescribing physician. Seek medical advice before stopping any medication or changing the way you take the drug.

10-POINT HOLISTIC TREATMENT PLAN FOR DEPRESSION

1. Identify and address any underlying organic or physiological cause of depression.
2. Develop a positive, optimistic mental attitude.
3. Increase the level of humor and laughter in your life.
4. If you smoke, get help to quit.
5. Avoid alcohol and stimulants, including caffeine.
6. Exercise regularly.
7. Perform a relaxation/stress reduction technique for ten to fifteen minutes each day.
8. Eat a healthy diet and take appropriate nutritional supplements.
9. Take appropriate doses of 5-HTP.

10. If necessary, supplement 5-HTP with L-tyrosine or D,L-phenylalanine, or with *Ginkgo biloba* or St.-John's-wort extract.

Remember Linda, my piano-playing patient? I had suggested that she try taking 5-HTP at a dosage of 150 mg per day. When she dropped by my office not long ago, I almost didn't recognize her. Her face was vibrant. Her mouth no longer bore that tight, pursed expression but a confident, winning smile. And her eyes had lost that glazed and puffy look. Now they sparkled with energy and joy.

Recalling our previous conversation, I asked her again what it was that she found pleasurable in her life. "Being alive," she answered. "Waking up after a good night's sleep. And being able to whip through that Bach piece as easily as 'Chopsticks.'"

Are You Depressed?

One effective way that doctors can assess the state of a person's moods and gauge the response to treatment is through the use of self-assessment questionnaires. These tests examine a number of areas in a person's life that can be affected by depression. Taking the same test several times over a period of weeks or months shows the underlying patterns of the illness and indicates if, and how, therapy is working.

If you think you are suffering from one of the forms of depression, complete the following checklist of symptoms, developed by the National Mental Health Association. This checklist will not diagnose depression; only a qualified medical professional can do that. But it will give you a general idea about the state of your mood.

Clinical Depression Checklist

Use the following checklist to determine if you or someone you know is suffering from clinical depression. If five or more of the following symptoms have lasted for more than two weeks, tell a doctor as soon as possible.

_____ Feelings of sadness and/or irritability

_____ Loss of interest or pleasure in activities once enjoyed

_____ Changes in weight or appetite

_____ Changes in sleeping pattern

_____ Feeling guilty, hopeless, or worthless

_____ Inability to concentrate, remember things, or make decisions

_____ Fatigue or loss of energy

_____ Restlessness or decreased activity

_____ Thoughts of suicide or death

_____ TOTAL

In addition, look for the following symptoms of the manic phase of manic-depression:

• Increased energy and decreased need for sleep

• Inappropriate excitement or irritability

• Increased talking or moving

• Promiscuous sexual behavior

• Disconnected and racing thoughts

• Impulsive behavior and poor judgment

Source: National Mental Health Association; used by permission.

Caution!

One of the most disturbing symptoms of depression is an overwhelming feeling of guilt, hopelessness, or despair. As a consequence, many depressed people feel that life is not worth living. They are plagued by recurring, intrusive thoughts about death and suicide. Perhaps 15 percent of severely depressed individuals attempt to kill themselves. Tragically, many succeed.

If you are depressed and are contemplating suicide, please get help immediately. Call a local suicide prevention hotline or your local emergency system (dial 911).

There is hope. Depression *can* be treated. Life can be made worth living again.

Key Points of This Chapter

- Depression is a widespread and serious problem.
- Low serotonin levels are a main contributing factor in depression.
- Most standard antidepressant medications work by increasing the activity (but not the levels) of serotonin and other neurotransmitters.
- 5-HTP is a natural method for raising brain serotonin levels.
- Clinical studies show 5-HTP to be an effective antidepressant.
- 5-HTP is superior to L-tryptophan for treatment of depression.

- Research shows that 5-HTP produces results equal to those achieved with standard antidepressant drugs, including SSRIs such as Prozac, with a much lower level of serious side effects.

- Some people may need to supplement 5-HTP treatment with use of catecholamine precursors (such as L-tyrosine) or herbal medicines (such as St.-John's-wort extract).

- Attitude, lifestyle, and nutritional factors are important factors in depression and are part of a complete program of treatment.

- Before beginning any treatment for depression, consult your doctor and undergo a complete medical examination.

- To avoid "serotonin syndrome," do not take 5-HTP if you are taking (or have taken within the past four weeks) a prescription antidepressant, especially an MAO inhibitor, without consulting your physician.

- Do not stop taking or adjust dosages of any prescribed medication without first consulting your physician.

- Do not try to diagnose depression yourself; only a qualified medical professional can diagnose this condition.

CHAPTER 3

5-HTP: THE NATURAL WEIGHT LOSS PRESCRIPTION

Several decades ago, researchers discovered that the serotonin system plays a major role in regulating your appetite. To be precise, it tells your brain that your hunger has been satisfied. As a result, serotonin puts the brakes on your food intake.

Since then, drug companies have been in a frantic race to come up with the "perfect" diet pill. Their most promising prescription medication for weight loss appeared to be fenfluramine, sold under the brand name Pondimin. Because fenfluramine tends to cause drowsiness, it was usually combined with an amphetamine-like drug called phentermine; the combination is known as "fen-phen." Later, scientists tinkered with the fenfluramine molecule and came up with a modified form, dexfenfluramine, better known as Redux. Redux went on sale in the United States in the summer of 1996.

But in September 1997 the news broke: Fenfluramine and its chemical cousin Redux pose a risk of life-threatening complications, including dangerously low blood pressure and permanent damage to the valves of the heart. The FDA urged people to stop taking the drugs immediately, and the company that sold the product, Wyeth-Ayerst, promptly recalled it from the market.

Fortunately, as you'll learn in this chapter, 5-HTP offers an alternative method of weight loss. Because 5-HTP boosts serotonin, it helps control hunger pangs. And 5-HTP has a key advantage over Redux and fen-phen: It is much, much safer.

Obesity and the Serotonin Connection

Surveys report that 30 percent of Americans, adults as well as children, are significantly overweight if not downright obese. Today, millions of people are struggling to lose weight in a safe, effective, and permanent way. Sadly, however, many of them are unable to achieve their goal. Despite popular belief, their failure is not because they lack the required desire or willpower. The problem instead is that they are trying to fight a war without a proper battle plan or access to effective weapons. Mounting evidence now shows that 5-HTP provides the ammunition that people need to win their "battle of the bulge."

Of course, no supplement can do the job all by itself. A complete natural program for permanent weight loss involves making significant changes in your diet and lifestyle. I'll briefly describe some of those steps at the end of this chapter.

But the promise of 5-HTP is that it makes these changes easier to achieve. That's because 5-HTP solves one of the biggest problems that contributes to obesity: serotonin deficiency. One important function of serotonin is to signal the brain when the body has eaten sufficient food. Scientists call this feeling of satisfaction the satiety mechanism. Because 5-HTP increases serotonin, and because serotonin makes you feel like you've eaten enough, taking 5-HTP reduces appetite. This means you take in fewer calories in the course of the day. Because serotonin also improves mood and raises your energy level, using 5-HTP also makes it much easier to stick to a diet and follow an exercise plan, which contributes further to weight loss. And 5-HTP lets you achieve these results without risking the dangerous—even deadly—side effects associated with synthetic drugs such as Redux and fen-phen.

Researchers have found that when animals and humans are fed diets lacking in the amino acid tryptophan, their appetite—the desire to eat—increases significantly. This in turn triggers bouts of binge eating—periods in which enormous amounts of food are consumed in a short period. During binges, people typically crave foods that are high in carbohydrates, such as sugars and starches. Experiments on animals also show that carbohydrates are the preferred item on the binge menu, but the animals will wolf down whatever food happens to be lying around.[1]

A diet low in tryptophan leads to low brain serotonin levels. Without enough serotonin, the brain senses that its metabolic needs are not being met and it responds as it would if it were actually starving. At that point the brain goes into the metabolic equivalent of "red alert." In an act of self-preservation, the brain sends out powerful signals to the appetite control centers. These signals tell the body: "Start eating fast—and if possible, stock up on carbohydrates."

There are two logical reasons for this. First, a carbohydrate-rich diet provides a quick source of energy to keep the body running. Second, a high-carbohydrate, low-protein meal increases the amount of tryptophan that is available to enter the brain through the blood-brain barrier (see Chapter 1, Figure 1.4). The more tryptophan in the brain, the higher the level of serotonin that can be manufactured. With more serotonin in circulation, the appetite regulation center receives stronger signals indicating that enough food has been consumed. This, in turn, switches off the food cravings . . . at least temporarily.

Low serotonin levels lead to carbohydrate cravings, and high carbohydrate intake leads to obesity. These cravings are also a key symptom of the eating disorder known as bulimia, which I'll talk about later in more detail.

Dieting only makes the problem worse. As several studies have demonstrated, dieting causes concentrations of tryptophan in the bloodstream—and consequently brain serotonin levels—to plummet.[2] Again, in response, severe drops in serotonin levels cause the brain to send out powerful and irresistible signals to eat. No wonder most diets don't work! The very act of dieting tells the brain to signal the body to start eating again. From the brain's point of view, dieting is a threat to its very survival.

In summary, most people trying to lose weight are fighting a battle they simply cannot win. Currently, over half of the adults in this country are trying to lose weight, but less than 5 percent of them—fewer than one out of twenty—will even come close to achieving the results they seek. However, bringing 5-HTP to the battle can mean the difference between crushing failure and resounding success.

5-HTP and Appetite

Back in the early 1970s, researchers conducted experiments on rats that had been genetically bred for obesity—in other words, fat rats. In addition to their bigger bodies, these rats also showed decreased activity of the enzyme that converts tryptophan into 5-HTP and ultimately into serotonin. Without this enzyme, the body and the brain can't whip up a fresh batch of serotonin to replenish the dwindling supply. As a result, these rats never get the message to stop eating—not, that is, until after they have consumed amounts of food that are far greater than those eaten by normal rats. The researchers found that giving 5-HTP to these rats resulted in significant drops in the amount of food the animals consumed.[3]

As you probably know, a lot of circumstantial evidence exists to suggest that some of us humans are genetically programmed to be obese. But what does this really mean? What message do these "obese genes" send out to the body? Animal studies such as the one I just described may provide the answer. It appears that in some cases obesity may result, at least to some extent, from a defect in the genes responsible for cranking out the enzymes we need to convert tryptophan to 5-HTP. Genetic problems are complex, and it isn't always possible to point to a single gene defect and identify it as the sole cause of a disorder. But in those cases

where a person's body is biologically unable to make enough serotonin, obesity can be one of the consequences.

That's another reason 5-HTP is such an exciting supplement.
Taking doses of 5-HTP means you can bypass any existing genetic
defect in your tryptophan enzyme factory. In other words, you
don't need the missing enzyme to make 5-HTP; you can take
5-HTP directly in the form of a supplement. 5-HTP is a shortcut
that saves steps and makes it easier for your body to produce the
serotonin you need to turn off the brain's hunger signals.

Do You Crave Carbohydrates?

Low serotonin levels trigger increased consumption of food in
general. People with a serotonin deficiency often experience cravings to eat large quantities of foods high in carbohydrates.

Carbohydrates come in two main varieties, simple and complex. Simple carbohydrates—sugars—are composed of one or two
sugar molecules. Foods high in simple carbohydrates include
candy, white bread, pastries, and most processed breakfast cereals. Complex carbohydrates—starches—contain many simple sugars joined together by chemical bonds. Foods rich in complex
carbohydrates include whole grains, pasta, and starchy vegetables
such as potatoes. People who have carbohydrate cravings will eat
carbohydrates in any form, but they strongly prefer the simple
sugars.

In severe cases, carbohydrate cravings develop into a kind of
addiction. The body gets caught up in a vicious dietary cycle: low
serotonin triggers overwhelming hunger urges; the urges cause
increased intake of carbohydrates; carbohydrates boost serotonin
levels quickly but temporarily; when the levels fall, the cycle begins again.

To determine if you are addicted to carbohydrates, take the
following quiz. The more yes answers you give, the more intense
your addiction—and the better your chances that 5-HTP will help
you control your cravings and lose weight.

Carbohydrate Addiction Quiz

_____ I get tired and/or hungry in the mid-afternoon.

_____ I crave bread, pasta, cereal, candy, and other carbohydrate-rich foods.

_____ When I start eating starches, snack foods, or sweets, I have a hard time stopping.

_____ After eating breakfast, even if it is a large satisfying meal, I get hungry before lunch.

_____ I am overweight.

_____ My body fat is primarily distributed around my abdomen and upper body.

_____ If I do not eat every two or three hours during the day, I feel tired, shaky, and irritable, and sometimes I develop a headache.

_____ I have one of the following health conditions: elevated cholesterol or triglyceride levels, diabetes, high blood pressure, hypoglycemia.

_____ I eat more when I am stressed or depressed or when I am traveling.

_____ I tend to gain more weight or have trouble losing weight in the winter months.

Scoring:

Number of Yes Answers	Extent of Carbohydrate Addiction
8–10	Severe
5–7	Strong
2–4	Mild to moderate
0–1	None

Bulimia: An Extreme Form of Carbohydrate Addiction

Cravings for carbohydrates can range in intensity from mild (occasional strong desires to nibble on a piece of bread or a cookie) to severe (prolonged bouts of uncontrollable eating known as binges). In many cases, people who binge-eat become overwhelmed with fear, guilt, and self-hatred, feelings that arise in part because of their eating habits. As a result, they may take extreme measures to get rid of the food. For example, they may induce vomiting by making themselves gag or by using an emetic drug known as ipecac. Many people with the disorder also take high doses of laxatives to cause food to leave the body more quickly, before the calories (and, for that matter, the nutrients) have time to be absorbed. These actions are known as purging. People who binge without purging are said to have a binge eating disorder. Those who binge and purge have bulimia (or, more technically, bulimia nervosa).

Interestingly, most people with bulimia are of normal weight. But as you can imagine, this binge-and-purge cycle wreaks havoc on the body. The medical consequences of bulimia can be quite severe, ranging from rupture of the stomach, erosion of the dental enamel from the acid contained in vomit, and problems with muscles—especially the heart—due to loss of potassium and other vital chemicals known as electrolytes. In severe cases, bulimia can be fatal.

Shockingly, bulimia is a relatively common condition, affecting approximately four out of every one hundred women. (Some men are also bulimic, but the rate of the disorder among males is much lower.)

Over the past two decades, evidence has accumulated supporting the idea that low brain serotonin levels are a major factor in bulimia.[4] An interesting study in this area was conducted a few years ago at the University of Pittsburgh School of Medicine.[5] The goal of the study was to measure the effect of lowered brain serotonin on food intake levels and on mood. The researchers enrolled ten normal-weight women with bulimia and ten healthy women matched for age and weight. The women with bulimia had not taken any medications to treat their bulimia for at least four weeks. Both groups of women then ate a specially prepared diet that omitted foods containing tryptophan; as I noted earlier, such a diet will result in reduced levels of serotonin. The results confirmed what the scientists predicted: The women with bulimia experienced increased food intake, irritability, depression, disorganized thinking, hunger, and urges to binge.

Based on the results of such studies, many researchers are now convinced that bulimia results when low serotonin levels trigger episodes of binge eating, especially of carbohydrates (Figure 3.1). The binges, in turn, lead to a flurry of serotonin production and release within the brain. High levels of serotonin then reduce—at least temporarily—the feelings of stress and tension. This serotonin "fix," however, is short-lived; it is usually followed by overwhelming feelings of guilt and low self-esteem, which can trigger a powerful desire to get rid of the food by purging. Low serotonin levels appear to be responsible for some of the personality traits commonly seen among people with bulimia, such as depression, impulsiveness, irritability, and emotional volatility.[6]

In treating bulimia, some physicians prescribe serotonin-active drugs such as Prozac. At the time this book is being written, no reports have been published in the medical literature specifically looking at the role of 5-HTP in the treatment of bulimia. There is some preliminary evidence that 5-HTP may be useful.[7] However, because of what we know about the effects of 5-HTP on the serotonin system, and because of my professional experience with the product, I am convinced that 5-HTP is a rational choice and an effective natural alternative for people with this disorder. Over the past few years I have treated perhaps a dozen bulimic women with 5-HTP and have seen very good results. Let me tell you about one of these cases.

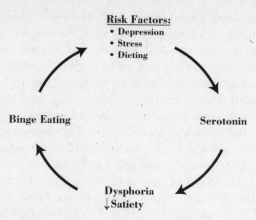

Figure 3.1: The Bulimic Cycle

Curing Carbohydrate Cravings:

JESSICA'S STORY

To judge from her school pictures, Jessica at age fifteen was a real dynamo. An attractive, active kid with curly brown hair and sparkling eyes, she was a member of the cheerleading squad and served on the student council.

But now, at age seventeen, she was a different person, barely recognizable. Her face was sallow and she had dark rings around her eyes. Her smile had faded into a fixed flat line. Once, her eyebrows had angled upward like accent marks, reflecting her optimistic and enthusiastic attitude. Now they tilted downward, giving her a constant look of fear and worry.

She didn't come to my office on her own accord. Her mother brought her to me out of a desperate awareness that her precious daughter was in deep trouble.

As I asked Jessica about her situation, I realized that she was a girl in tremendous turmoil. She had been battling bulimia for nearly a year. Almost every other day she experienced severe carbohydrate cravings. Her "drug of choice" was heavily sugared breakfast cereal, especially Cap'n Crunch. She told me she could gorge on two or three boxes of the stuff at a time. "Usually," Jessica said in an unexpressive voice, "I just go into the bathroom, stick my finger down my throat, and throw it all up again." The day before our visit, her mother had found her passed out on the bathroom floor.

Just a few weeks earlier Jessica had been discharged from an inpatient treatment center, where she had taken part in an intensive thirty-day program. Her doctors had prescribed Zoloft, a serotonin reuptake inhibitor, but she said it made her feel agitated and nauseated and she stopped taking it. She was participating in individual therapy twice a week. Because bulimia is often considered a family problem—tensions and struggles at home can stir up emotions and control issues that can trigger episodes of bingeing and purging—her family was also seeing a counselor.

Despite these measures, Jessica still felt her life was out of control. Her marks in school had plummeted, she had withdrawn from most of her activities, and she had recently broken up with her boyfriend. "The only man I'm seeing much of these days is the guy they call Cap'n," she said dryly. Since none of the other treatments she tried were working, her mother suggested that Jessica consider an alternative approach to therapy. That's why they came to me.

I explained my perspective on bulimia to Jessica. I told her that it's a serious illness, very difficult to treat, because it affects both the body and the mind in a tangled pattern—like a dance with the devil. I described the serotonin system in simple terms and showed her how the emotional stresses she was experiencing in her life were affecting her brain's chemical balance and causing her to feel depressed. Depression was a result of decreased levels of serotonin. Without adequate supplies of this important chemical, her mood would remain flattened.

What's more, serotonin affects the appetite control center of the brain, especially those "switches" that tell her body when it's time to stop eating. The lack of a shutoff valve causes her to go on eating binges. Those binges make her feel more stressed out and depressed . . . and round and round we go. "We need to help you get off this not-very-merry-go-round," I told her.

I prescribed 100 mg of 5-HTP to be taken three times a day, twenty minutes before meals. I explained my hope that 5-HTP would raise her serotonin levels and curb her cravings. As an added measure, I asked Jessica to keep a diary in which she would record the food she ate, note and describe her food cravings, and describe her moods and thoughts about food. When her energy level returned, I hoped she would begin exercising regularly. I also made her promise to make a concerted effort to avoid high-sugar foods. "It's time you told the Cap'n to sail off into the sunset," I said. At this remark, I saw her give the first faint hint of a smile.

Jessica came to my office a week later. She said that she had noticed results with 5-HTP almost immediately. By the fourth day, she said, she was feeling more in control, had fewer and less intense food cravings, and was sleeping better. "I just feel . . . I don't know, *lighter*," she said. At the time this book was written, Jessica had been following the 5-HTP regimen for three months. She remained in good spirits, and with one exception has had no episodes of bingeing and purging.

As is true of the struggle to overcome other forms of addiction, battling carbohydrate cravings can be a lifelong battle. Since low serotonin levels may be the result of a chronic, possibly genetic, deficiency, it is likely that Jessica will be on 5-HTP for a very long time, perhaps indefinitely. "I can deal with that," Jessica told me during our last session. "I'd rather swallow a 5-HTP pill than another box of that godawful cereal."

5-HTP as a Weight Loss Aid

One of the most promising roles for 5-HTP is in helping people lose weight. Early animal studies with 5-HTP were followed up by a series of three human clinical studies conducted at the University of Rome's Internal Medicine Department under the direction of Carlo Cangiano and Fabrizio Ceci. I'd like to discuss the findings from these studies in detail to explain how 5-HTP works so effectively as a weight loss agent.

All three studies assessed patients using a tool called the body mass index, or BMI. Body mass is a better way of analyzing health risks than simply measuring weight. The BMI gives us a general idea of the amount of fat your body contains, and indicates whether the body mass is appropriate for a person's height. BMI is calculated by dividing your body weight in kilograms divided by your height in meters squared. To figure those values in the more familiar English system, first divide your height in inches by 39.4 and multiply the result by itself. This gives you your body area in square meters. Then divide your weight in pounds by 2.2 to get your weight in kilograms. Then divide your weight by your height and there you are: your BMI value.

Body Mass Index (BMI) Calculation

1. Convert weight in pounds to kilograms:
   Weight (in pounds) _____ divided by 2.2 = _____ kg
2. Convert height in inches to meters:
   Height (in inches)___ divided by 39.4 = ___ meters
   Square the meters (Multiply value in meters by itself):_____ × _____ = _____
3. Calculate BMI
   Divide weight in kg __ by meters squared __ = __
4. Your BMI: _____

If you haven't converted to the metric system and you don't have a calculator handy, I'll make it easier for you. Just consult the BMI table on page 112 (Figure 3.2).

Height*

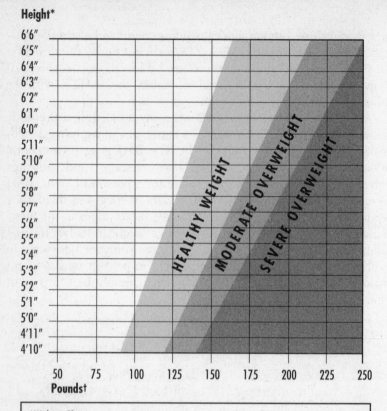

*Without Shoes.
†Without Clothes.
Source: Report of the Dietary Guidelines Advisory Committee on the Dietary Guidelines for Americans. 1995, pages 23-24.

BMI	Health Risk
Under 25	Very Low
25-30	Low
30-35	Moderate
35-40	High
Over 40	Very High

Figure 3.2: BMI Table

5-HTP and Obesity: Study #1

The first Italian study involved nineteen overweight female subjects with a body mass index ranging between 30 and 40.[8] To give you an idea of how significant these women's weight problems were, a typical woman who is 5'4" and whose BMI is 30 would weigh 170 pounds; a woman that tall with a BMI of 40 would tip the scales at around 235 pounds. Ideally, a 5'4" woman should weigh between 110 and 145 pounds. As you can see, these study subjects were significantly obese. Depending on how you calculate it, these women were anywhere from 15 percent to more than 100 percent over their desired body weight. More practically speaking, they were, on average, 30 to 80 percent heavier than they should be.

Before the treatment phase of the study began, the scientists analyzed the women's dietary intake. They concluded that the patients' main problem was that they ate too many carbohydrates. They also asked the women to fill out food diaries for three days at the beginning of the treatment period and again at the end. During the study, their food was carefully weighed before the meals; any leftovers were reweighed so the researchers knew exactly how much they had eaten. Twice a week the participants also filled out a self-evaluation of appetite and satiety. Their mood was evaluated as well, using standard psychological tests.

The researchers then gave the patients daily doses of 5-HTP. The study dose was 8 mg per kilogram (2.2 pounds) of body weight, or approximately 200 mg three times per day. This was a placebo-controlled crossover study. (For more information on what these terms mean, see Chapter 2.) In one phase, patients took either the 5-HTP or a placebo twenty minutes before meals for five weeks. After a one-week interval during which no treatment was given, the patients were crossed over to the other treatment. (That is, the ones who received 5-HTP in the first phase started taking placebo, and vice versa.) The women were then allowed to eat the way they normally would. The researchers put no restrictions on their diet, because they wanted to find out whether 5-HTP reduced appetite and promoted weight loss without any conscious effort on the part of the patient.

The results of the study were nothing short of incredible. Table 3.1 shows the sharp declines in the subjects' intake of calories, protein, and carbohydrates.

Table 3.1: 5-HTP and Obesity Study #1:
Effect of 5-HTP and Placebo on Food Intake

	Food intake (calories/day)	Protein Intake (g/day)	Carbohydrate Intake (g/day)
Prior to treatment	2,903	101	274
Placebo	2,327	85	223
5-HTP	1,819	79	176

While taking 5-HTP, the women consumed nearly 1,100 fewer calories per day—a decrease of more than one third, or about 37 percent. The average amount of weight loss during the five-week period of 5-HTP supplementation was a little more than three pounds. In contrast, during the placebo period, they lost only about one pound of total weight. The drop in calories was due mainly to their reduced intake of carbohydrates, which fell by a similar proportion.

Let me put these exciting results into perspective. A person who reduces calories to that extent would burn off about one and a half pounds of fat each week, six pounds in a month, and *a whopping seventy-three pounds in a year.*

Remember, too, that these impressive results were achieved even though the women did nothing else to their diet. They did not *consciously* reduce food consumption or increase their daily exercise.

The self-tests that the women took showed that there were no differences in their appetite (their degree of hunger just before they started eating) during the two phases. The main difference occurred in their level of *satiety,* the satisfied feeling that comes from having eaten enough. In other words, 5-HTP did not reduce appetite before a meal, but after the women had consumed an adequate amount of food (a lesser amount than they would otherwise eat), the satiety centers in the brain were stimulated and the women no longer felt hungry. As a result, their caloric intake fell dramatically.

Following a policy of "trust but verify," the researchers confirmed that the patients actually took the doses of 5-HTP by conducting urine tests that measured the level of the serotonin breakdown product, 5-hydroxy-3-indoleacetic acid (5-HIAA). The tests showed that levels of 5-HIAA during 5-HTP treatment increased over fiftyfold compared with the control group. Besides confirming that the patients were indeed taking the 5-HTP, the increase clearly indicated that 5-HTP increased the levels of serotonin in the body.

5-HTP and Obesity: Study #2

How effective is 5-HTP in helping overweight people stick to a diet? To answer that question, the Italian research team recruited fourteen overweight female subjects with a body mass index ranging between 30 and 40 (again, roughly 30 percent to 80 percent above their ideal body weight) for a double-blind study.[9] As in the previous study, analysis of diets showed that these women were overweight, not because of a fundamental metabolic problem such as a glandular disorder, but because they tended to overeat, especially carbohydrates. The women were randomly assigned to receive either 5-HTP (300 mg three times a day, for a total daily dose of 900 mg) or a placebo thirty minutes before meals. Neither the patients nor the researchers knew which patients were taking the active treatment. By coincidence, the average weight among women assigned to the 5-HTP group was higher than that of women in the placebo group.

The twelve-week study involved two phases. For the first six weeks, the women had no dietary restrictions; they could eat any amount of any food they chose. In the second phase, however, they were placed on a restricted 1,200-calorie-a-day diet. (A typical diet in the United States contains 2,000 to 2,500 calories per day.)

Every two weeks the women came to the clinic, where the researchers evaluated their body weight, diet diaries, and self-evaluations of appetite and satiety. The women were also asked if they experienced such symptoms as changes in their sense of taste or smell, early satiety (feeling full before the meal is over), and nausea or vomiting. As before, urine tests verified that they were taking 5-HTP.

Did these women lose weight while taking 5-HTP? You bet. Over the course of twelve weeks those taking a placebo lost an average of only 2.28 pounds (remember, they were on a low-calorie diet for half the time). In contrast, the weight loss among the 5-HTP group was an average of 10.34 pounds—nearly a pound a week.

Table 3.2: 5-HTP and Obesity Study #2:
        Effect of 5-HTP on Weight Loss

	Placebo	*5-HTP*
Average weight (pounds)		
Baseline	207.68	229.46
After 6 weeks	206.58	225.94
After 12 weeks	205.40	219.12
Total weight loss (pounds)		
After 6 weeks	1.10	3.52
After 12 weeks	2.28	10.34

The difference in the weight loss between the two groups was impressive. I must emphasize, too, that reducing caloric intake was a big factor in the results. During the "normal diet" phase, the women taking 5-HTP lost an average of about 3.5 pounds, while during the restricted-calorie phase their loss nearly doubled, to about 7 pounds.

According to the urine tests, the level of 5-HIAA among the 5-HTP group increased by 60 times, from a pretreatment average of 8.8 mg per day to 501 mg per day, reflecting the dramatic increase in serotonin levels. In contrast, among the placebo group, the average level of 5-HIAA actually dropped a bit, from 7.3 to 6.9 mg per day. This drop may have been due to the fact, mentioned earlier, that dieting reduces tryptophan levels and consequently lowers serotonin, which in turn reduces levels of 5-HIAA in the urine.

As in the previous study, the researchers concluded that 5-HTP promoted weight loss by promoting early satiety, which every woman taking 5-HTP in this experiment reported. Some of the women also stated that during treatment they began developing an aversion to meat or they noticed changes in their sense of taste and smell (Table 3.3). (Perhaps the increase in serotonin had something to do with these changes; the study is not very specific on these points.)

Table 3.3: 5-HTP and Obesity Study #2: Reported Effects

	5-HTP		Placebo	
	Week 1–6	Week 7–12	Week 1–6	Week 7–12
Taste alteration	2/7	1/7	0/7	0/7
Smell alteration	2/7	1/7	0/7	0/7
Meat aversion	3/7	1/7	0/7	0/7
Early satiety	7/7	6/7	2/7	2/7
Mild nausea	5/7	0/7	1/7	2/7

As the table shows, five out of the seven women receiving 5-HTP in this study experienced mild nausea during the first six weeks of the trial. In Chapter 2, I explained that some people experience this side effect as a normal and temporary reaction to increased serotonin levels. The relatively high incidence among this small group may have to do with the fact that higher doses of 5-HTP (900 mg per day) were used in this study. After six weeks on 5-HTP, however, none of the women complained about nausea, while some of the women on placebo did. In my practice, I have found several methods for helping patients control the mild transient nausea that sometimes arises during the first few weeks of therapy with 5-HTP. (See the recommendations for the use of 5-HTP in depression in Chapter 2, page 76).

5-HTP and Obesity: Study #3

More evidence in support of 5-HTP as a weight loss aid comes from a well-designed double-blind study conducted at the University of Rome.[10] As in the previous studies, this one enrolled overweight women with carbohydrate cravings and BMIs between 30 and 40. The twenty-eight subjects received either 5-HTP (300 mg three times daily before meals, total daily dose 900 mg) or a placebo. For the first six weeks there were no dietary restrictions, and for the second six weeks the women followed a diet that supplied 1,200 calories per day, distributed as follows: Carbohydrates contributed 53 percent of the calories, fats 29 percent, and proteins the remaining 18 percent. During this phase no carbohydrate-rich snacks were permitted between meals. The subjects were examined every two weeks to evaluate food intake and body weight. Routine blood measurements were also performed at the beginning, at six weeks, and again at the end of the study. To verify patient compliance with the 5-HTP treatment, urine tests for 5-HIAA were conducted.

The results from this study were even more impressive than the previous studies for several reasons. The group receiving 5-HTP lost an average of 4.39 pounds within the first six weeks and an average of 11.63 pounds after twelve weeks. In compari-

son, the placebo group lost an average of only 0.62 pounds after
the first six weeks and 1.87 pounds after twelve weeks. The lack of
effective weight loss among those receiving a placebo prompted
researchers to question the subjects further. They found that the
women in the placebo group clearly had a tough time sticking to
the restricted-calorie diet. "Why bother avoiding food," they
seemed to be saying, "if I don't see any results?" In contrast, the
women taking 5-HTP had a much easier time following the restricted diet.

Table 3.4: 5-HTP and Obesity Study #3:
Effect of 5-HTP on Weight Loss

	Placebo	*5-HTP group*
Weight (pounds)		
Baseline	207.46	219.34
After 6 weeks	206.84	214.95
After 12 weeks	205.59	207.71
Total weight loss (pounds)		
After 6 weeks	0.62	4.39
After 12 weeks	1.87	11.63

An average weight loss of nearly one pound per week, regardless of the reason, is exceptional. In this study, as in the others
discussed here, the researchers attributed the weight loss from
5-HTP to increased serotonin levels, which caused early satiety
and led to decreased overall food intake. Early satiety was reported by 100 percent of the subjects during the first six-week
period. During the second phase, even with severe caloric restriction, 90 percent of the women taking 5-HTP continued to report
early satiety. In other words, even though they were eating less,
they still felt full. As in the previous study, most of the 5-HTP
group reported mild nausea during the first six weeks of therapy.
However, the symptom was never severe enough to cause any of

the women to drop out of the study. No other side effects were reported.

The use of 5-HTP apparently made it easier for the treated patients to stick to their low-calorie diet in the second phase of the study. Generally, the reduced calories were the result of cutting down on carbohydrate-rich foods. (Remember, the study was conducted in Rome, where traditional lunches and dinners include pasta followed by a protein source and lots of bread.)

Back in the Swing:

CATHY'S STORY

Cathy is a fifty-six-year-old woman who came to see me for help with her golf game. Well, indirectly, at least.

The problem wasn't her inability to keep the ball from slicing. Her real handicap was that although she stood only 5'1" in her stocking feet, she weighed in at 160 pounds. According to the BMI charts, she was about twenty-five pounds overweight. Not that those excess pounds necessarily kept her from the golf course. But in Cathy's case, her weight was putting excessive strain on her knees and contributing to a serious problem among women her age: osteoarthritis. This form of arthritis is the most common, and it causes destruction of cartilage in the joints. Cartilage is like a soft, spongy cushion. It protects the ends of joints by acting as a shock absorber. Degeneration of the cartilage is the hallmark of osteoarthritis, leading to severe joint pain and restricted movement. In Cathy's case, her bum knees were ruining her once-glorious pendulum swing.

Carrying around excess pounds greatly increases your risk of developing osteoarthritis in weight-bearing joints such as the knees, hips, and spine. If Cathy hoped to ease her pain, I told her, she needed to lose some weight.

But when we started talking about this problem, Cathy became very upset. She told me how frustrated and embarrassed she was by her ballooning figure. All her life, until now, she had been very fit and active. She attributed her previous ability to maintain her body weight to the fact that she golfed two to four times a week. Most of the time she walked the course, using a cart only if her partner was unable to keep up with her.

In the past few years, though, her weight had started becoming a problem. She had gained twenty-six pounds in two years. In other circumstances I might simply have shrugged off her weight gain as a by-product of her advancing age and the fact that she had started taking hormone replacement therapy to treat symptoms of menopause. But as a concerned physician—and a curious person—I probed a little deeper.

Cathy told me that the needle on the scale had started inching upward during the months following her mother's death. As part of my routine examination, I asked her if anything ever made the weight gain problem better, and she replied, "Sure—whenever I can get in a round of eighteen holes." What made it worse, she said, was when her knees were so sore that she couldn't hobble around the fairways.

I asked what she thought was responsible for her gain. In my experience, I've found that patients often have the right clues to their condition, if you're smart enough to let them tell you.

"I always seem to be hungry," Cathy replied. "It doesn't matter how much I eat, I never really feel satisfied. And I feel . . . I don't know, kind of blue all the time."

Her comment raised a red flag in my mind. I thought about the scientific reports I'd tucked away in my files about the effect of serotonin on the satiety signals, those appetite-regulator pathways in the brain. I remembered, too, the comments by Dr. Judith Wurtman in her book *The Serotonin Solution* about how stress— such as the death of a loved one—can trigger a domino effect, in which emotional turmoil can lower serotonin levels.

At first glance Cathy's case seemed fairly straightforward. In clinical practice, though, things are rarely cut-and-dried. Sensing that the loss of her mother had been devastating, I spent about a half-hour out of our forty-five-minute session probing more deeply about the special bond they enjoyed. "She was my best friend," Cathy said. During our talk, I learned that her mother had been a rich source of nurturing in her life. Cathy loved her husband and two grown sons. "After Mom died they said and did all the right things," Cathy said, "but they simply were not able to fill that void I felt in my life—a void I still feel to this day."

I suggested that Cathy try to develop some other strategies to help get the nurturing she clearly needed. In this way she would be less likely to overeat as a way of trying to compensate for what was lacking in her emotional life. As we chatted, Cathy commented that she loved playing golf not so much because she enjoyed the game—although she did—but rather because she enjoyed being with her golfing-buddy girlfriends. Her weight, and the burgeoning problems with arthritis, were robbing her not just of the pleasure of the game but of the pleasure of her friends' companionship.

I urged Cathy to cut out refined sugars and increase the fresh vegetables in her diet. I recommended a high-potency multivitamin and increased doses of vitamins E and C for optimal nutritional support and to increase her levels of antioxidants. I also recommended 5-HTP plus *Ginkgo biloba* extract to address her moods, reduce her carbohydrate cravings, and readjust her satiety signals.

I also suggested that she try glucosamine sulfate to help with her osteoarthritis. Glucosamine is a nutrient substance that the body combines with other proteins to create cells that make up the cartilage, nails, tendons, skin, bones, ligaments, and heart valves. Taking glucosamine can increase the strength and integrity of joints and the tissues that hold them together. When sufficient levels of glucosamine are present, cartilage better retains its ability to hold water and act as a shock absorber. This naturally occurring compound is better than anti-inflammatory drugs in the treatment of osteoarthritis, and it does not cause side effects.[11] The standard dosage of glucosamine sulfate is 500 mg three times daily. As a final suggestion to Cathy, I recommended that she find other activities that she could enjoy with her circle of friends—playing cards, going to movies or museums—at least until her other problems eased up.

Cathy came in for her return office visit six weeks later. In that time she had lost eight pounds. "At this rate, the treatment is going to cost me a fortune in new clothes," she said happily. The constant hunger she had experienced for the past couple of years had vanished. Her arthritis was still troubling her, but she noticed the first glimmerings of improvement. She had been able to go golfing a couple of times—"although I had to ride in that darn cart," she complained—and she was noticeably thinner and much more alive and vibrant.

At the six-month mark Cathy had lost those twenty-six extra pounds, and another four for good measure, and she was pain-free. She agreed with my suggestion that she could probably stop taking 5-HTP and glucosamine sulfate but that she should continue with the other supplements. Her reduced weight and the improvement in her arthritis have brightened her outlook and brought her a higher quality of life.

During Cathy's last visit, her only complaint was that there was no natural treatment known that would help her reach a coveted goal: making a hole-in-one.

Why Isn't There More Research on 5-HTP?

The results from the three clinical studies at the University of Rome demonstrate that 5-HTP offers tremendous benefits as a weight loss aid. But this raises a question: Why isn't there more research in this area? To answer the question, it helps to remember the slogan of the investigative reporter: "Follow the money."

As a rule, medical research is sponsored by pharmaceutical companies, which naturally hope to reap huge financial rewards from their discoveries. Basic research, such as the research conducted on serotonin and eating behavior, often focuses on natural compounds found in the body, such as tryptophan and 5-HTP. After these biochemical processes have been identified, research shifts to a search for drugs that alter those body processes—drugs that can be patented, protected, and sold exclusively by the company that developed them. With a natural, nonpatentable substance such as 5-HTP, there is little financial incentive for researchers to invest hundreds of thousands of dollars and years of study. Such research will not produce a patentable product, and consequently the costs of research will not be recouped. In contrast, developing a unique and patentable drug can make millions for the discoverers, the research institutions, and the pharmaceutical companies.

As you can imagine, this situation means that sometimes new drugs appear on the market that aren't necessarily better than natural, unpatented alternatives but that have a lot more scientific research to support their use.

5-HTP vs. Redux

There is no doubt that the diet drugs Redux and fen-phen worked. Doctors wrote millions of prescriptions for the drugs, and millions of people lost millions of pounds. Unbeknownst to patients and their doctors, however, nearly one in three of them was also losing something else: normal, healthy heart valve tissue. I'll discuss the safety issue in a moment. First, though, let's take a quick look at how 5-HTP compares in efficacy with the diet drugs.

Like 5-HTP, Redux inhibits appetite and promotes weight loss by increasing the effects of serotonin on appetite control centers in the brain. Redux does so in two ways: by increasing the manufacture and release of serotonin from the neuron, and by blocking the reuptake of serotonin, much like the SSRI antidepressants such as Prozac. (For more information about this process, see Chapters 1 and 2.) In contrast, 5-HTP has only one mechanism of action: It raises serotonin levels but does not block reuptake.

Results from a one-year study conducted at various medical centers in Europe in the late 1980s suggested that Redux worked . . . but not all that well.[12] Known as the International Dexfenfluramine (INDEX) Trial, the study enrolled 822 patients. One group received Redux (dexfenfluramine), 15 mg twice daily, and the other received a placebo. Because this was a double-blind study, neither the researchers nor the patients knew who was receiving the active drug. Over the course of a year, the dexfenfluramine group lost an average of twenty-one pounds—just five pounds more than the average sixteen pounds lost by patients in the placebo group, who, remember, were taking an inactive "dummy" pill.

Of the 822 patients who began the study, only 518 completed it. The dropout rate in the dexfenfluramine group was 37 percent, while in the placebo group it was 45 percent. Among the placebo group, the high rate of dropout was attributed mainly to a dissatisfaction with the rate of weight loss. Among the dexfenfluramine group, dissatisfaction was also a problem, but many of the patients also cited problems with serious side effects, such as fatigue, diarrhea, dry mouth, increased urinary frequency, and drowsiness. About one person in three taking the active drug complained of side effects.

Interestingly, virtually all of the weight loss reported in the INDEX Trial occurred within the first six months. Most of the people in the dexfenfluramine group actually regained two to four pounds during the second half of the year, even though they were still taking the drug. Apparently, then, Redux lost its effectiveness over time.

This underscores another advantage of 5-HTP: Its ability to

help you lose weight, or maintain your desirable weight, continues throughout the course of therapy. In my practice, I have found that patients can keep taking 5-HTP for as long as they need to reach their weight loss goal. They do not start regaining weight, even after six months or more of 5-HTP therapy. It appears that, over time, increased serotonin levels resulting from 5-HTP actually reset the appetite control centers in the brain. The result is decreased appetite. This allows patients to eventually stop taking 5-HTP without fear that lost weight will return. Of course, they need to take additional steps to keep weight off, such as exercising and eating a reduced-calorie diet.

To compare the effects of 5-HTP with those of Redux, there should be direct head-to-head comparisons. However, no such comparative studies have been published. The best we can do is compare the results of separate studies.

Earlier I described results of the Italian studies, which examined the ability of 5-HTP to reduce patients' calorie intake. A similarly designed study with dexfenfluramine was conducted at four major university hospitals in the Netherlands.[13] The subjects, men and women with a body mass index between 28 and 35 (roughly 25 to 40 percent above their ideal body weight), received either dexfenfluramine (30 mg/day) or a placebo for nine weeks. Compared to the placebo, dexfenfluramine led to a reduction in calories consumed and significant weight loss. The average weight loss during the nine weeks was about 6.5 pounds in the dexfenfluramine group; the placebo group had no weight loss. These results are slightly better than the 3.2 pounds lost during five weeks of 5-HTP treatment and the 3.52 and 4.39 pounds lost after six weeks in the other two studies. The average rate of weight loss without dietary restrictions is roughly 0.72 pounds per week with Redux versus 0.65 pounds per week with 5-HTP—a difference of about 1.3 ounces, or the weight of a snack-size bag of potato chips.

In other words, the difference between Redux and 5-HTP in terms of weight loss is not very impressive.

Let's now take a look at the difference between Redux and 5-HTP when people follow a restricted diet. In double-blind studies where Redux (30 mg per day) was used along with caloric restriction (1,200 calories per day for women; 1,500 calories per day for men), researchers found that the average total weight loss after twelve weeks was a little less than eleven pounds.[14] This rate of loss is very close to the level achieved with 5-HTP (10.34 pounds in study #2 and 11.63 in study #3). Remember, though, that in the 5-HTP studies, there were *no dietary restrictions* during the first six weeks.

The Redux Risk

But efficacy is not the most important issue. As I said, Redux works. But as patients have discovered, the price, in terms of life-threatening side effects, was too high to pay.

Even before Redux came on the market, scientists knew that it and fenfluramine could cause a life-threatening condition known as primary pulmonary hypertension. This problem causes changes in the blood vessels in the lungs, resulting in slower blood flow (in medical terms, increased resistance). Blood can't reach the lungs as easily, which causes the lungs to fail, thus starving the rest of the body of the oxygen it needs to function. During treatment with Redux or fen-phen, primary pulmonary hypertension would strike apparently healthy individuals within the first two months of therapy. Primary pulmonary hypertension can be fatal. Some people die very soon after the condition develops; overall, one out of four will die within two to five years. Taking these drugs for longer than three months greatly increases the risk.

Primary pulmonary hypertension resulting from these drugs affected between eighteen and forty-six of every million users, or less than one person in sixty thousand. In the medical world, that qualifies as a "rare" complication. In its review of the scientific data, the FDA agreed that the health benefits of weight loss offset the possible risk from primary pulmonary hypertension. Even so, had Redux and fenfluramine not been withdrawn, the rapidly growing popularity of these drugs would undoubtedly have led to a significantly higher number of cases of—and more deaths from—primary pulmonary hypertension.

What led to the withdrawal of these drugs, however, was not a rare complication but a dangerously frequent one. In the summer of 1997, researchers at the Mayo Clinic reported that people who were taking fen-phen had waxy deposits that coated their heart valves.[15] Other investigators spotted the problem in patients taking Redux.[16] The valve defect shows up on echocardiograms. Over time, the deposit can become so thick that it can prevent the valve from closing properly. When that happens, the heart may not be able to generate enough pressure to keep the blood flowing through the vessels properly. Heart valve disease is a silent killer; it often does not cause any symptoms, so people are unaware that they are in danger. But the danger is real: In time, the valves can fail, leading to death. Responding to the Mayo study, the FDA ordered further tests at five other clinics. Researchers found valve abnormalities in 92 out of 291 patients—over 31 percent—who had taken fenfluramine or Redux. When these results came in, the FDA concluded that the drugs posed an "unacceptable risk" and the drugs disappeared from the market. As this book was being written, further studies were under way to assess the extent of the damage.

In addition to the life-threatening heart valve problem, Redux causes troublesome side effects in another one out of three patients. The most common complaints include insomnia, which occurs in 20 percent of people who use the drug, diarrhea (17 percent), headache (16 percent), weakness (16 percent), dry mouth (12 percent), increased urinary frequency (2.8 percent), and drowsiness (7 percent). In contrast, 5-HTP does not cause these side effects. In double-blind studies on 5-HTP as a weight loss aid, some patients complained of mild nausea during the first few weeks of therapy, but the problem was so mild that none of the patients stopped using the substance.

At the very least, lacking direct head-to-head comparisons, we can conclude that 5-HTP promotes weight loss about as effectively as Redux and with fewer serious side effects.

If Redux, fenfluramine, and 5-HTP all increase serotonin levels, wouldn't 5-HTP pose the same danger to heart valves? There are no published clinical reports to indicate that such is the case. Unlike Redux, 5-HTP does not block reuptake of serotonin. And unlike the MAO inhibitors, 5-HTP does not interfere with the activity of the enzyme that breaks down serotonin. The point here is that 5-HTP does not disrupt the normal process of serotonin release, reabsorption, and elimination from the body. Besides, 5-HTP is not a synthetic drug; it is an amino acid produced naturally by your body's metabolism. In contrast, some pharmacologists have referred to Redux as a "dirty" drug because of its adverse and unintended effects in the body.[17]

The problems associated with excess serotonin can arise from two major causes: the presence of tumors that release serotonin (known as the carcinoid syndrome), or the effects that develop when a serotonin-active antidepressant (an SSRI or tricyclic) is taken in combination with an MAO inhibitor.[18] People with carcinoid tumors are known to be at higher risk of heart valve disease. But scientists have been unable to induce valve disease in experimental rats by injecting them with high doses of serotonin on a daily basis.[19] As I interpret these findings, the danger from serotonin-producing tumors comes not from the serotonin itself, but from increased levels of other substances the tumors produce. Among these substances are the kinins, which cause inflammation. Chronic inflammation due to the presence of kinins can lead to tissue breakdown and can damage heart valves.

As for the problem caused by combining antidepressants: the use of tricyclics or SSRIs at the same time as an MAO inhibitor is absolutely contraindicated. Warnings to this effect appear in all the literature that accompanies these drugs. I have conducted a careful search of the scientific data and have turned up no reports of heart valve disease or other problems related to serotonin syndrome in people who take 5-HTP by itself.

Of course, we all benefit from ongoing scientific research that aggressively examines these questions. I hope that, as more people become aware of the potential benefits of 5-HTP, more studies will be done to assess its safety and efficacy on an ongoing basis. Meanwhile, having prescribed 5-HTP for hundreds of patients, I can continue to recommend it as a safe and effective product that provides numerous benefits, including weight loss.

Enhancing the Weight Loss Benefits of 5-HTP

If you are serious about losing weight, taking 5-HTP alone is not enough. For best results, you also have to make some profound changes in your lifestyle. Even though the $4-billion-a-year weight loss industry does its best to convince you otherwise, no pill exists that will end your weight worries immediately and forever. Ask anyone you know who was able to lose weight and then keep it off. Odds are that the person succeeded by changing their dietary and living habits. 5-HTP can help this process by providing valuable support.

Why are so many Americans overweight? The answer is simple: Each day they consume more calories than they burn off in physical activity. If you want to lose weight, you need to take in fewer calories while burning off excess calories at a faster rate. In other words, eat less, exercise more.

Each pound of fat contains about 3,500 calories. If you want to lose a pound a week, you need to have a "negative calorie intake" of 500 calories a day—that is, you must burn 500 more calories than you consume. You can achieve this by reducing the number of calories in your diet, by exercising more, or both. 5-HTP helps reduce the intake of calories by switching on your satiety signals.

You need a certain number of calories for your body to function normally. To determine your caloric needs and choose an appropriate target for weight loss, you must identify your ideal weight. Of course, "ideal" is relative. A person with a small body frame will weigh less than a person with a large frame, even though their height may be the same. So step one is to determine your frame size (see box on page 131).

Body Frame Size

Place a ruler on a table. Then extend your arm and bend the forearm upward at a 90-degree angle. Keep the fingers straight and turn the inside of your wrist away from your body. Using your thumb and index finger of your other hand like calipers, measure the distance between the two prominent bones on either side of your elbow. Without changing the distance between your thumb and index finger, measure the gap against the ruler. Find the measurement listed on the following table and look at the top of the column to determine whether you have a small, medium, or large frame. For example, if you are a woman 5′4″ in height and your elbow breadth is 2⅜″, you have a medium frame.

Table 3.5: Determining Your Frame Size

	Height	Elbow Breadth (inches)		
		Small Frame	Medium Frame	Large Frame
Men	5′2″ to 5′3″	<2½″	2½″–2⅞″	>2⅞″
	5′4″ to 5′7″	<2⅝″	2⅝″–2⅞″	>2⅞″
	5′8″ to 5′11″	<2¾″	2¾″–3″	>3″
	6′0″ to 6′3″	<2¾″	2¾″–3⅛″	>3⅛″
	Over 6′4″	<2⅞″	2⅞″–3¼″	>3¼″
Women	4′10″ to 5′3″	<2¼″	2¼″–2½″	>2½″
	5′4″ to 5′11″	<2⅜″	2⅜″–2⅝″	>2⅝″
	Over 6′0″	<2½″	2½″–2¾″	>2¾″

< = less than; > = greater than

Now look at Table 3.6 to determine your ideal body weight for your frame size. For example, according to this table, a hypothetical woman five feet six inches tall with a small frame should weigh between 120 and 133 pounds. This chart was originally developed by the Metropolitan Life Insurance Company back in the early 1980s. It's not perfect, but at least it gives you a rough idea. Talk to your doctor or other health care professional to learn what weight is right for a person of your age, physical condition, and overall health.

Table 3.6: Metropolitan Life Height and Weight Table

| | Height (ft/in)° | Weight (lbs)° | | |
		Small Frame	Medium Frame	Large Frame
Men	5'2"	128–134	131–141	138–150
	5'3"	130–136	133–143	140–153
	5'4"	132–138	135–145	142–156
	5'5"	134–140	137–148	144–160
	5'6"	136–142	139–151	146–164
	5'7"	138–145	142–154	149–168
	5'8"	140–148	145–157	152–172
	5'9"	142–151	148–160	155–176
	5'10"	144–154	151–163	158–180
	5'11"	146–157	154–166	161–184
	6'0"	149–160	157–170	164–188
	6'1"	152–164	160–174	168–192
	6'2"	155–168	164–178	172–197
	6'3"	158–172	167–182	176–202
	6'4"	162–176	171–187	181–207
Women	4'10"	102–111	109–121	118–131
	4'11"	103–113	111–123	120–134
	5'0"	104–115	113–126	122–137
	5'1"	106–118	115–129	125–140

5'2"	108–121	118–132	128–143
5'3"	111–124	121–135	131–147
5'4"	114–127	124–138	134–151
5'5"	117–130	127–141	137–155
5'6"	120–133	130–144	140–159
5'7"	123–136	133–147	143–163
5'8"	126–139	136–150	146–167
5'9"	129–142	139–153	149–170
5'10"	132–145	142–156	152–173
5'11"	135–148	145–159	155–176
6'0"	138–151	148–162	158–179

° Weights for adults age 25 to 59 years based on lowest mortality. Weight in pounds according to frame size wearing indoor clothing (5 pounds for men and 3 pounds for women) and shoes with 1-inch heels.

Source: Metropolitan Life Insurance Company, 1996; used by permission.

Okay, break out the calculator. Now we're going to determine your daily calorie needs. First, convert your ideal weight in pounds to kilograms by dividing the number by 2.2. Next, multiply that by the following "calorie constant" according to your overall activity level:

Little physical activity: 30 calories
Light physical activity: 35 calories
Moderate physical
activity: 40 calories
Heavy physical activity: 45 calories

Weight (in kg) × Activity Level = Approximate Calorie Requirements

_____ × _____ = _____

The woman in our hypothetical example has an ideal body weight of about 125 pounds, or 57 kilograms. She is moderately physically active; she exercises about half an hour every other day and works at a desk job. Her calorie constant is 40. Thus her calorie requirement is 57 × 40, or 2,280 calories a day.

Naturally, people are eager to lose weight as quickly as they can. My recommendation, though, is to set a moderate goal of an average of one pound of fat loss per week. Losing two pounds a week runs the risk that you will lose muscle tissue, not just fat. Crash diets and quick weight loss programs ultimately fail because they slow down your metabolism and cause loss of muscle. In the long run, the tortoise will always beat the hare.

I suggest setting a goal of taking in 250 fewer calories than your approximate calorie requirement, as calculated above. This will promote weight loss and still provide you with the energy you need to function. Additional calories can be burned through other means, including exercise.

Approx. calorie requirement _____ − 250 = Calorie target _____

For our hypothetical woman, her target caloric intake is 2,030 (2,280 − 250).

Other Aspects of a Complete Weight Loss Program

Before undertaking a weight loss regimen, you should talk to a medical doctor, naturopathic physician, nutritionist, or other health care professional who has a special interest in nutrition. These people can help design a program that is right for your individual needs. Meanwhile, here are some general guidelines that will help.

GET EXERCISE

Someone once said, "The best exercise you can do is to push yourself away from the dinner table." That's partly true; eating less helps. But increasing your activity level provides many benefits in addition to shedding a few pounds. Besides burning off excess calories, exercise strengthens the heart, improves circulation, prevents bone loss, and helps fend off a number of serious diseases and disorders. Exercise must be a part of an overall weight loss plan for a number of reasons (see box below).

The Importance of Exercise in Weight Loss

- Weight lost through dieting only comes from loss of muscle tissue and water weight.
- Exercise improves the ratio of muscle to fat. Since muscle burns calories while fat stores calories, an increase in muscle mass means your body burns more calories more efficiently, all day long—even while you're asleep.
- Dieting alone reduces your basal metabolic rate (BMR), the rate at which your body burns calories when you are inactive or at rest. Adding exercise prevents this drop in the BMR.
- Increased metabolic rate (and calorie burning) continues for a period of time even after the exercise session is over.
- Exercise enhances mood and self-esteem; moderate to intense exercise also helps suppress your appetite.
- Exercise helps you maintain weight loss over time.

Of course, most people find it very hard to develop an exercise routine and stick to it. Talk to your health care professional and find out what kind of exercise program is right for you. Whatever you do, remember that exercise is absolutely essential for health.

As a rule of thumb, doing exercise that boosts your heart rate for about thirty minutes a day is a reasonable and healthy goal to shoot for. Construct a daily diary and checklist. It always helps to see your progress in black and white. Keep track of your dietary habits, your exercise routines, and other important information. Also note what positive affirmations you made each day. Some people use these diaries to keep lists of things they are grateful for. For more tips, see the box, Seven Steps to Successful Exercise, below.

Seven Steps to Successful Exercise

1. *Realize how vital exercise is to your health.*
2. *Consult your physician before beginning.* This is especially important for people over age forty or for anyone who is out of shape or who has a history of heart disease, smoking, high blood pressure, dizziness, fainting spells, or irregular heartbeat.
3. *Select an activity you enjoy.* If you hate jogging, then you won't be motivated to stick to the plan. On the other hand, if you love walking, then let that be your exercise of choice. Walking briskly (four or five miles per hour) for forty-five minutes will burn off 250 calories. Aerobic exercise—which increases heart rate—is important. So is weight training, in which you exercise specific muscles by lifting or moving weights. Weight-bearing exercise is important for preventing bone loss due to osteoporosis. Increasing muscle mass increases the rate at which your body burns calories.
4. *Monitor exercise intensity.* To find the ideal "training zone" for your heart rate during exercise, subtract your age from 185. If you are forty years old, your maximum heart rate should be 145. Subtract

another 20 to get the bottom of this exercise range. Thus a forty-year-old person should exercise so that the heart rate stays between 125 and 145 without going over the maximum. You need to sustain this rate for at least twenty to thirty minutes to get the benefits of exercise.

5. *Do it often.* You don't get in good physical condition by exercising once a week. Exercise must be performed on a regular basis. For weight loss, you will want to work out at least five days a week. Exercising at the lower end of your training zone for longer periods of time is much better than exercising at a higher intensity for a shorter period of time.

6. *Use the buddy system.* People who have workout partners are more likely to stick to the program.

7. *Stay motivated.* Do whatever it takes to keep your enthusiasm level high:

- Read magazines to learn about new exercise plans and to remind yourself of the benefits of what you're doing.

- Set goals that are realistic so you don't feel discouraged.

- Vary your routine so you don't get bored.

- Record your progress in a diary so you can see how well you're doing.

- Join a health club. Having a facility with good equipment makes it easier to stay committed. The very act of paying for membership in a club helps many people exercise often so they can "get their money's worth."

FOLLOW A PROPER, DIET

Using 5-HTP is just one aspect of weight loss. Another crucial aspect is your diet. A complete guide to diet lies beyond the scope of this book. Briefly, though, here are some of the most essential dietary guidelines to help you lose weight and keep it off.

A diet does not necessarily mean reduced food intake. Instead, you should change the type of food you eat to reduce the calorie content and provide effective nutrition. This means choosing high-fiber, low-calorie foods, especially vegetables, legumes (beans), most fruits, and whole grains.

A good diet contains a mixture of carbohydrates, proteins, and fats. (Yes, you need some fat so that your body can produce healthy cells and tissues.) As a rule, the goal is to obtain your calories in the right ratio. Typically, that ratio is:

Calories from carbohydrates:	60 to 70 percent of total calories
Calories from fats:	5 to 25 percent of total calories
Calories from protein:	15 to 20 percent of total calories

In addition, you should consume between 35 and 50 grams of fiber a day.[20]

Do not skip breakfast. After a good night's sleep, you need to provide your body with food to get your physical and mental systems running. Choose whole-grain, high-fiber cereals (hot or cold) and consider using soy milk rather than cow's milk. Cow's milk is a common food allergen, and even in its low-fat form it can raise cholesterol levels. In contrast, soy foods offer protection against heart disease and certain forms of cancer (especially breast and prostate cancer). Avoid cereals with added sugar, and watch for hidden fat. Surprisingly, some granolas and other "natural" cereals are high in fat content.

For that matter, don't skip lunch, either. People who skip one or two meals and then gorge on a big dinner put too much of a metabolic load on their bodies all at once. The healthiest diet is one in which you eat several smaller meals throughout the day. Lunch is a great time to enjoy a healthy bowl of soup (especially one with beans or legumes, such as peas or lentils) and a large salad.

For dinner, the healthiest meals include a fresh vegetable salad, a vegetable side dish (steamed, baked, or boiled), and whole grains (in the form of bread or pasta). Legumes should be in there somewhere, either as an ingredient in soup or salad or as an entree, such as a bean casserole. Avoid starchy vegetables, such as potatoes. If you choose to eat meat or other animal products, limit your intake to no more than four ounces per day. Choose fish, skinless poultry, and lean cuts of meat.

Believe it or not, snacks are an important part of a diet. Eating the right snack at the right time can keep your energy level up. What's more, a snack can keep you from getting dangerously hungry, which in turn helps prevent you from overeating when mealtime finally comes along. The trick is to choose the *right* snacks. Fruits and vegetables—raisins, carrot sticks, cherry tomatoes, and so on—are best. A few rye crispbread crackers, followed by a large glass of water, help fill your stomach and provide you with an extra smidgen of fiber. Air-popped popcorn (hold the butter!) is another good snack. Raw nuts and seeds provide protein, but many of them are also high in fat.

Treatment Recommendations for Weight Loss

In summary, here are my suggestions for using 5-HTP as part of your weight loss program.

Start by taking 100 mg of 5-HTP three times a day. Choose an enteric-coated form of the product, because these pills do not dissolve in the stomach. Instead, they pass into the small intestine, where the active ingredient is metabolized with a lower risk of nausea. Take the dose twenty minutes before your meals.

Stick with this approach for at least four weeks. If your weight loss results are unsatisfactory after that time, try doubling the dosage to 200 mg three times a day. Again, continue for at least a month. You should experience a weight loss averaging about one pound per week.

If you're not happy with your progress, it is possible to increase the dose to 300 mg three times a day, or a total daily dose of 900 mg. In my opinion, though, it is seldom necessary to take such high doses to achieve excellent results. I have not seen improved weight loss when my patients take 900 mg of 5-HTP per day compared to 600 mg. If after trying the lower doses you increase the level and your rate of weight loss improves, then great. If you don't notice any difference, however, I suggest going back to a regimen of 200 mg three times per day. Never take more than 900 mg of 5-HTP a day for any reason.

Under no circumstances should you begin your 5-HTP treatment at the higher dosage levels. There is no added benefit in doing so and there is a risk of more severe nausea. By gradually increasing the dosage of 5-HTP over the course of two months or more, you have a much better chance of preventing nausea from becoming a problem.

Be sure to follow the additional recommendations presented in this chapter to promote safe and effective weight loss.

Key Points of This Chapter

- Most attempts to lose weight fail because they do not address the basic underlying problem: an imbalance in serotonin, the brain chemical that regulates appetite and triggers feelings of fullness and satiety.

- Low brain serotonin levels promote carbohydrate cravings and overeating.
- Human obesity may be caused in part by faulty serotonin synthesis.
- Bulimia (binge eating, or the binge-and-purge cycle) is linked to low serotonin levels.
- 5-HTP addresses eating problems by boosting serotonin levels.
- 5-HTP has proved useful in reducing food cravings in many people, including those who have bulimia.
- Studies show that 5-HTP reduces calorie consumption and promotes weight loss.
- Redux and fenfluramine, diet drugs that promoted weight loss by affecting the serotonin system, were pulled from the market when it was found that they posed an unacceptably high risk of life-threatening complications, including primary pulmonary hypertension and heart valve disease.
- 5-HTP used alone is not associated with serious adverse effects.
- 5-HTP should be used in conjunction with a complete program that includes exercise, a healthy mental attitude, and a proper diet.
- Start by taking the lowest recommended doses of 5-HTP for weight loss, 100 mg three times a day. If results are unsatisfactory, wait at least four weeks before increasing

the dose to 200 mg three times a day, and another four weeks before increasing to the maximum dose, 300 mg three times a day.

- To reduce the risk of nausea, take the dose of 5-HTP twenty minutes before meals.

CHAPTER 4

5-HTP AND THE TREATMENT OF INSOMNIA AND OTHER SLEEP DISORDERS

A good night's sleep is one of the most precious gifts we humans can enjoy. Sound, restorative sleep is the foundation of a healthy life. Of course, sleep provides the rest your body needs. Just as important, sleep is vital for healthy brain activity during the day. You need to sleep deeply and restfully—and, what's more, you need to dream—so that your moods, emotions, reflexes, and cognitive ability can function at their best during your waking hours.

But for many people, getting a good night's sleep is something that, if you'll excuse the expression, they can only dream about. At some time in their lives, around seventy million Americans will experience insomnia or some other sleep disorder. For 60 percent of these, the problem is chronic. The overall toll exacted by this situation, which some experts refer to as "sleep debt," is enormous: higher incidence of physical diseases, mood disorders, bone-aching fatigue, reduced ability to maintain and nourish healthy relationships with friends and family members, and loss of a sense of joy in just being alive.

Perhaps it will come as no surprise to learn that the complex biological process we call sleep depends to a great extent on a healthy, well-functioning serotonin system. Research shows that serotonin is vital for helping us fall asleep. Serotonin also helps us stay asleep, especially during the early phases of the sleep cycle, before we enter the dream stage. (I'll say more about the sleep cycle in a moment.) Finally, serotonin serves as a kind of chemical coordinator, a hormone that regulates the production and activity of other hormones involved in sleep. Not surprisingly, then, sleep disorders are among the most common and devastating consequences of the serotonin deficiency syndrome.

In my years of experience treating thousands of patients who suffer from a variety of complaints, I have come to believe that addressing sleep disorders is the single most important step I can take. Good sleep is the wellspring from which flow all other benefits—increased stamina, resistance to disease, slower aging process, elevated mood.

The most common form of sleep disorder is insomnia—the inability to fall asleep and stay asleep throughout the night. A number of natural and herbal medicines are available for the treatment of insomnia. Among the most well known are melatonin and valerian. In my view, however, 5-HTP provides the quickest, most effective, and most consistent overall results. In virtually every case where I have prescribed 5-HTP, it has worked to improve my patients' sleep quality. Clinical studies are also showing that 5-HTP produces promising results in the treatment of sleep disorders other than insomnia. This chapter will highlight the importance of 5-HTP as a good alternative to prescription and over-the-counter sleeping pills.

Sleep Patterns

Human sleep is perhaps one of the least understood biological processes. Surprisingly, scientists aren't even sure why we need to sleep. Recently, though, researchers at Stanford University may have found an answer, and it has to do with the brain and its energy supply. In order to function, the brain can burn only glucose, the main form of sugar found in the body. Your muscles also use glucose. If your glucose supply drops too far, your muscles can also burn fat to make up the difference, but your brain can't burn fat. Instead, your brain will tap into the energy stored inside cells in the form of another sugar known as glycogen. Before it can raid the glycogen cupboard, however, the brain has to release a substance called *edenizine,* which brings on sleep. Thus sleep takes place because your brain needs to build up its energy level, and the only way it can do so is when you are inactive and asleep. In a sense, the brain needs to shut down a few of its circuits so it can upgrade its energy supply.

The consequences of inadequate sleep can be dangerous— even deadly. Research has found that healthy men deprived of even a single night's sleep have a 30 percent drop in the activity of their immune system's tumor-fighting cells the next day. The electrical activity in the brain during dream sleep puts a stop to muscle activity, which allows the body to reconstruct damaged muscle tissue. Lack of sleep deprives your body of the time it needs to repair worn-out tissue. Research has also found that people who get only four and a half hours of sleep in a night experience a surge of high blood pressure when they awaken in the morning. In some cases, that surge can lead to stroke or other heart problems. Sleep problems add nearly $16 billion to the nation's total costs for health care each year.

According to the U.S. Department of Transportation, each year two hundred thousand sleep-related accidents claim more than five thousand lives (other experts put the number at closer to twenty-three thousand deaths). Accidents caused by sleepy drivers also produce hundreds of thousands of injuries. Shockingly, a survey of physicians found that 42 percent of them admitted that they had caused the death of at least one person because they had been too sleepy to make wise medical decisions or perform surgery properly.

How much sleep do you need? That depends on who you are. Individual sleep needs vary greatly. Many people can get by on five or six hours a night. Others need nine or ten hours. There is no fixed formula.

Generally, though, and up to a certain point, sleep needs decrease with age. A one-year-old baby requires about fourteen hours of sleep a day. By age five, children need about twelve hours. Adults, on average, need about seven to eight hours. Women tend to require more sleep than men. As you may be aware, many elderly people do not sleep as long at night as their younger counterparts. It is a myth, however, that elderly people "need" less sleep. Their sleep requirement—seven or more hours a night—remains about the same as it was in younger adulthood. What changes with age, however, is the person's ability to *sustain* sleep effectively. There are many reasons for this, but one crucial factor is the decreased efficiency of serotonin system function in the aging brain. The elderly tend to sleep less at night but doze more during the day than younger adults. A better approach is to facilitate sound, consistent sleep during a single nighttime session.

Scientists study sleep patterns using a machine called an *electroencephalograph,* or EEG. This devices measures brain wave patterns during sleep. Over the decades, researchers have identified a clear pattern, or "architecture," of normal sleep. Distinct variations in this pattern occur in the different sleep disorders.

Basically, sleep occurs in a series of cycles, each lasting between sixty and ninety minutes. A normal sleep pattern involves four to seven such cycles during the course of the night. On average, people have five or six sleep cycles during a normal nighttime sleep session.

Each cycle has two main parts. During the first part, our level of consciousness falls while the level of unconsciousness rises. This part of the cycle involves changes in heart rate and breathing, and an overall slowing of brain activity. We do not dream during this phase. In the second part of the cycle, however, we do dream. The characteristic sign of this phase of sleep is rapid eye movement, or REM.

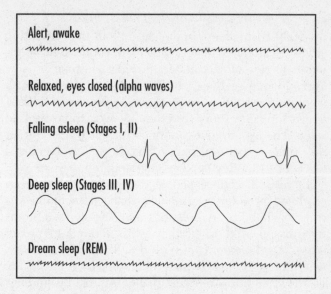

Figure 4.1: Brain Waves During Sleep

The Importance of Dreams

The author Anatole France wrote, "Existence would be intolerable if we were never to dream." I believe this statement to be profoundly true.

A dream is a sequence of sensations, images, and thoughts passing through a sleeping person's mind. A dream can also present in our waking hours as a wish, fantasy, desire, or fanciful vision. It is our dreams that propel us through this life. They are powerful, inspirational, and potentially healing.

Scientific proof of the importance of dreams can be found by studying the negative effects in people who are prevented from dreaming—that is, who are deprived of REM sleep. In the early 1960s the pioneering sleep researcher William C. Dement conducted experiments in this subject at Mount Sinai Hospital in New York. In one of these studies, subjects sleeping in a laboratory setting were awakened the moment REM began to occur; they were then allowed to go back to sleep. The experiment continued for one week. During this time the test group reported greatly increased levels of irritability, anxiety, and appetite.

In related studies, people deprived of REM sleep exhibited profound personality changes, including extreme irritability, depression, and anxiety, symptoms that disappeared when they were allowed to dream again.[1] Dr. Dement later moved to Stanford University, where he participated in several studies on the ability of 5-HTP to improve sleep quality. Among his findings was that 5-HTP increases REM sleep significantly (typically by about 25 percent) while simultaneously increasing deep sleep stages 3 and 4 without increasing total sleep time.[2]

Some experts believe that all of us dream, even if we don't remember dreaming. If you feel you do not dream, or if you want to enhance the vividness of dreams and your ability to recall them, you may need some help from 5-HTP to get you started. Of all the roles that 5-HTP can play, the one that I use it for most often is to promote sleep and, consequently, to improve dreaming. I often recommend 5-HTP to patients if they tell me that they do not remember their dreams, even if they do not complain of insomnia per se.

Generally, then, each ninety-minute sleep cycle contains a non-REM period (also called slow-wave sleep) and the REM period.

On average, each of these two main periods occupies about 50 percent of the cycle's elapsed time, or about forty-five minutes. In fact, however, the balance between the two periods shifts during the course of the night. During the first ninety-minute cycle, the REM phase might last only a few minutes. In the final cycle of the night, REM sleep occupies most of the time, perhaps an hour or more.

Non-REM sleep actually consists of four distinct substages, labeled 1 through 4. The stages are defined according to the types and intensity of brain wave activity as measured by EEG tracings, and also by the ease with which the sleeping person can be aroused. As you no doubt know, if you have just dropped off to sleep, you can usually be easily awakened quickly with full awareness of where you are and what's happening. The deeper you get into the non-REM stages, however, the harder it is to become aroused. You might wake up and perform some activity, such as going to the bathroom or even holding a brief conversation with your bed partner. But the odds are you won't recall doing so in the morning.

When you enter the REM stage, however, your brain suddenly becomes much more active. After the flurry of REM activity subsides, brain wave patterns will return to non-REM sleep stage 1, and another ninety-minute cycle begins. One of the key differences between the phases is that people aroused during non-REM sleep will not recall having any dreams. They might report thoughts, such as a list of things they have to do the following day, but not dreams. In contrast, people aroused during the REM stage are usually able to report that they were dreaming, and they can often recall their dreams in great detail.

As people age, they tend to spend less time in the REM stages. What's more, many people tend to wake during the phase of transition out of non-REM into REM sleep. Such nighttime awakenings, of course, lessen the beneficial effects of sleeping. As a consequence, people who suffer from this form of sleep disturbance often wake in the morning feeling groggy and unrested, and they continue feeling fatigued throughout the day. This problem, also known as fragmented sleep, is common among the elderly and other people who suffer from chronic serotonin shortage.

Taking 5-HTP, however, helps to "smooth out" the rough spots in the sleep pattern, preventing this arousal during transitional phases and promoting deeper, more restful sleep. This was shown in a study conducted at Stanford on alcoholics who were trying to overcome their addiction.[3] Their long-term use of alcohol had resulted in very fragmented and unrestful sleep, as measured by disturbances in their REM-stage sleep. But when they took oral doses of 5-HTP, most of them slept much better. EEG tracings showed that the improved sleep resulted from less fragmented REM cycles. In this group of patients, the more severe the sleep problem, the better their response to 5-HTP. The researchers concluded that 5-HTP corrects the serotonin deficiency that leads to sleep problems. In my view, this benefit is one reason why my elderly patients and others with serotonin deficiency do so well on treatment with 5-HTP.

Insomnia and Drug Treatment

At some point during the course of a year, about half the U.S. population will have difficulty falling asleep. For one person in three, insomnia occurs on a regular basis. About 17 percent of the population reports that insomnia causes major problems in their lives: daytime fatigue, irritability, trouble functioning on the job.

Understandably, people with insomnia are desperate for relief. Many use over-the-counter sedatives, while others—over eleven million a year—seek stronger prescription medications from their physicians. So-called hypnotic drugs—those that induce sleep—are among the most widely used of all medicines. The hypnotics include sedatives, minor tranquilizers, and antianxiety drugs. Doctors write thirty million prescriptions a year for sleeping pills and tranquilizers, and Americans spend more than $200 million annually on these products. If you were to pile together all the prescription and over-the-counter drugs used to help Americans sleep in the course of a single year, they would tip the scales at over 600 tons!

Sleep aids, both OTC and prescription varieties, are usually effective in the short term. That is, they work for about three or four days. They can help you get past a temporary disturbance in your normal sleep pattern, such as during travel or while you are recovering from an illness.

For simple insomnia, the medications most prescribed by doctors are the hypnotic drugs known as *benzodiazepines*. About 60 percent of prescriptions for sleep medicines are for drugs of this type. The benzodiazepines are generally regarded as the least dangerous of the hypnotics. However, they can still lead to potentially severe problems, such as changes in brain cells. These changes can show up as severe memory impairment and amnesia (forgetfulness), especially for events that occur while under the influence of the drug. Other adverse reactions include nervousness, confusion, hallucinations, bizarre behavior, and extreme irritability and aggressiveness. Overdose can lead to coma and malfunction of the heart and breathing systems (cardiorespiratory collapse). In some cases, especially if the sleeping pill is combined with alcohol, use of these drugs has proved fatal. Benzodiazepines have also been shown to increase feelings of depression, including suicidal thinking.

Another class of hypnotics is the *barbiturates*. Until the availability of benzodiazepines, these were the most commonly prescribed hypnotics. However, barbiturates are highly addictive and they pose a great risk of coma or lethal overdose, especially if combined with alcohol. These drugs can rob you of the restful deep non-REM and REM sleep stages. Withdrawal from the medications can cause REM rebound (excessive, overactive dreaming), hallucinations, anxiety, and, in severe cases, seizures. The barbiturates most commonly prescribed for sleep are secobarbital (Seconal), amobarbital (Tuinal), and pentobarbital (Nembutal). However, treatment of sleep problems with barbiturates is on the wane; only about 5 to 10 percent of prescriptions for sleep medications involve use of these drugs.

Tricyclic antidepressants are also prescribed for sleep. They are often useful if the insomnia causes you to wake up too early in the morning, a common symptom of serious depression. The most sedating of the antidepressants are *amitriptyline* (Elavil) and *doxepin* (Sinequan). Paradoxically, other tricyclics such as *protriptyline* and *desipramine* can be stimulating. Imipramine is sometimes used in the treatment of sleep-related problems such as sleepwalking and bed-wetting. Like barbiturates, tricyclic antidepressants can suppress REM sleep. Side effects include severe dry mouth, sweating, constipation, and heart problems such as abnormal heartbeat (arrhythmia). Tricyclics can interfere with the effects of medications taken to lower blood pressure, and they can lead to daytime drowsiness.

The most common OTC medication for sleep is an antihistamine called *diphenhydramine* (Benadryl). Another antihistamine, *doxylamine,* is an ingredient in a few OTC sleep aids, but evidence of its safety is not well established. Some OTC sleep aids also include a pain reliever, such as acetaminophen. Side effects of antihistamines include confusion, light-headedness, dry mouth, constipation, difficulty with urination, and blurred vision. The elderly are more prone to experience these problems.

Over-the-counter sleeping pills are generally less dangerous than prescription medications, but they can also interfere with normal sleep patterns. And they affect your coordination and reflex responses as well. As little as 50 mg of Benadryl may impair your ability to drive as severely as if you had a blood alcohol content of 0.1 percent, the standard for drunk driving.[4]

Paradoxically, some prescription sleeping pills can even make insomnia worse by interfering with the normal architecture of sleep and causing a type of "hangover" in the morning. The main reason is that these drugs disrupt both the REM-phase sleep and the non-REM deep sleep stages (stages 3 and 4). The sleep that results from use of sleeping pills tends to occur at a very superficial level. Such light sleep provides little in the way of benefit to the body or mind. Unless you experience appropriate deep sleep and dream sleep that is adequate in terms of both the number and duration of REM phases, you are likely to wake up feeling more tired than when you went to sleep. In contrast, 5-HTP actually *enhances* both REM and the deep-sleep stages. By raising serotonin levels, 5-HTP provides more of the fuel your brain needs to regulate sleep activity.

People taking prescription and OTC sleeping pills often get caught up in a vicious cycle. They take the drug, which does induce sleep but which also disrupts the quality of sleep throughout the night. In the morning, they wake up unrefreshed and groggy. In an attempt to get going, they typically drink large quantities of coffee. High levels of caffeine further disrupt the ability to fall asleep, leading to increased use of the sleeping aid . . . and so on and so on.

These drugs can also produce a phenomenon known as *tolerance*. That means your body gets used to having the drug, forcing you to take increasingly higher doses to achieve the same benefits as when you first started taking it. Tolerance in turn makes these drugs habit-forming—many people feel they have to keep taking them just to stay "normal." Often when you stop taking hypnotics you experience withdrawal symptoms, including rebound insomnia (return of insomnia in a more severe form) and increased anxiety. In addition, hypnotics can be physically addictive, not just psychologically habit-forming. It is possible to take a dangerous, even fatal, overdose of these medications. Hypnotics can suppress the breathing control center of the brain, leading to breathing cessation. This is a special danger in the elderly. They also cause drowsiness and reduced daytime alertness. If you take a hypnotic at the same time as other drugs, such as antihistamines, narcotics, alcohol, or antidepressants, the risk of these complications is much higher.

Trying to wean yourself off the medications can complicate matters. When you withdraw from long-term use of prescription sleeping pills, your REM sleep stage goes through a kind of "rebound" period. It becomes abnormally long or intense. Other symptoms of withdrawal from prescription sleep aids include anxiety, irritability, sensations of panic, insomnia, nausea, headache, impaired concentration, memory loss, depression, extreme sensitivity to the environment, seizures, hallucinations, and paranoia.

It's enough to keep you awake at night.

Fortunately, there's a safer and equally effective alternative natural approach: 5-HTP.

Warning

If you have been taking a prescription sleeping pill for more than four weeks, do not stop taking the drug suddenly. Talk with your physician about ways to taper off the drug gradually. Doing so helps you minimize or avoid potentially dangerous withdrawal symptoms.

Addressing the Causes of Insomnia

In most cases, insomnia is a symptom of a deeper problem or underlying physical disorder. Treating insomnia without looking for and addressing its real cause is like trying to fix a broken pipe by mopping up the floor. You may clean up some of the mess, but you aren't doing anything to stop the flood.

Effective treatment of insomnia only occurs after you and your medical care provider identify and address its true cause. In the overwhelming majority of cases, insomnia arises from a psychological problem, such as depression, anxiety, stress, or tension. Common physical causes include various medical disorders (see box on page 155), certain foods or drinks, and the use of certain medications. (There are more than three hundred prescription drugs on the market that list sleep disturbance among their potential side effects!)

Medical Causes of Sleep Problems

- Cardiac conditions
  Angina
  Arrhythmia
  Atherosclerosis (hardening of the arteries)
  Congestive heart failure
  High blood pressure
- Endocrine disorders
  Hormonal fluctuations of menstruation, pregnancy, or menopause
  Overactive thyroid
- Gastrointestinal conditions
  Colitis
  Enteritis
  Heartburn (gastroesophageal reflux)
  Irritable bowel syndrome
  Peptic ulcers
- Head and central nervous system problems
  Alzheimer's disease
  Degenerative conditions (such as Parkinson's disease or multiple sclerosis)
  Encephalitis (brain infection)
  Epilepsy
  Headaches (especially migraines)
  Hydrocephalus (fluid accumulation in the brain)
  Increased intracranial pressure due to ruptured blood vessel in the brain
- Respiratory conditions
  Asthma
  Chronic obstructive pulmonary disease

Sleep apnea
- Skeletal and muscle conditions
    Arthritis
    Pain
    Trauma or injury
- Other
    Hospitalization
    Rashes
    Recovery from surgery
    Sunburn

Source: Donald R. Sweeney, M.D., *Overcoming Insomnia: A Medical Problem for Problem Sleepers* (New York: Putnam, 1989).

Sleeping Soundly:

ANN'S STORY

Ann had a medical history consistent with serotonin deficiency syndrome. She was mildly depressed and a little overweight. She suffered from recurrent migraine headaches and said that she had received a diagnosis of fibromyalgia (chronic widespread body pain; see Chapter 6). Not surprisingly, Ann didn't sleep well. She woke up in the morning feeling exhausted. When she came to see me, she looked about ten years older than her real age of forty-two.

Her doctors had prescribed treatment with low doses of a tricyclic antidepressant, imipramine. She had taken the medicine faithfully for three months. While it had helped her mood a little, it did nothing to improve her sleep, and she still ached from the wracking pain of fibromyalgia.

I recommended 5-HTP, 100 mg three times a day, twenty minutes before meals, along with my baseline supplementation program of high-potency multiple vitamin and mineral formula, extra antioxidants, and flaxseed oil. For good measure, I recommended St.-John's-wort extract, 300 mg three times a day (see Chapter 7). In consultation with her doctor, Ann tapered off and finally discontinued the imipramine.

A few weeks went by, and Ann called to let me know that nothing much had changed. She was disappointed that this last ray of hope for treating her problem didn't seem to be working. I encouraged her to stick with the program, and explained that sometimes it takes a while for 5-HTP to restore serotonin and other transmitters, including pain-relieving endorphins, to the necessary levels.

At Ann's next checkup, three months into her therapy, she reported that she was "100 percent recovered" from the fibromyalgia. She was sleeping like a log and felt energetic and happy. Her appetite, especially for carbohydrates, was under control; she had lost ten pounds and expected to lose another ten. Ann's demeanor was so lively and enthusiastic that I look forward to seeing her when she returns for her six-month follow-up visit.

Experts have identified two main types of insomnia. *Sleep-onset insomnia* refers to difficulty in falling asleep, while *sleep-maintenance insomnia* refers to difficulty in staying asleep. Knowing which type is involved provides clues about the underlying cause (Table 4.1).

Table 4.1: Causes of Insomnia

Common Causes of Sleep-Onset Insomnia	Common Causes of Sleep-Maintenance Insomnia
Anxiety or tension	Depression
Environmental change	Environmental change
Emotional arousal	Sleep apnea
Fear of insomnia	Nocturnal myoclonus
Phobia of sleep	Hypoglycemia

Disruptive environment	Other forms of sleep disorder (parasomnias)
Pain or discomfort	Pain or discomfort
Caffeine	Drugs
Alcohol	Alcohol

The Problem with Prednisone:

JULIE'S STORY

My patient Julie is a clear example of how side effects of drugs can interfere with sleep. Julie is fifty-two years old and very petite—barely ninety-five pounds. She suffers from rheumatoid arthritis, and when she came to see me she was in a crisis. For several months she had been taking prednisone, a corticosteroid prescribed by her doctor. The drug relieved the pain and inflammation of her arthritis, but it also was causing depression and insomnia, side effects that occur in up to 57 percent of patients taking prednisone. By this point Julie looked beat. Her eyes were swollen with dark circles from lack of sleep. She said she really felt out of control and that she was too worn out to cope with her situation.

I explained to her that long-term use of prednisone was notorious for its severe adverse reactions, including increased appetite and weight gain and a risk of developing high blood pressure, ulcers, and other serious conditions. We worked out a program of natural remedies designed to address her arthritis. I also recommended that she try 5-HTP; because of her tiny frame, I felt the lowest dose (100 mg once a day at bedtime) would probably work for her. She was willing to do anything if it meant she could once again enjoy a good night's rest.

Well, just four days later we spoke by phone. She said that 5-HTP was "a life-saver." She was sleeping well and had noticed that her morning stiffness wasn't as bad. She agreed to talk to her doctor about weaning her off the prednisone and trying the alternative approach. When I last spoke to her, about six months into her program, she said she was sleeping like a baby and feeling on top of the world again.

Often the cause of the sleep disturbance involves an unhealthy lifestyle choice, such as poor diet or lack of exercise. If there is no medical problem involved, I always urge my patients to address these lifestyle issues before using any type of sedative product, including 5-HTP. Following are some of the important steps that can help you achieve natural, restorative sleep.

ELIMINATE SLEEP INHIBITORS

Your diet should be free of natural stimulants such as caffeine and its related compounds. Caffeine activates the nerves and muscles and stimulates the heart to get the blood flowing. In medicine, caffeine is used to treat migraine headaches, drowsiness, and mental tiredness. Too much caffeine causes such problems as racing heartbeat, stomach and bowel distress, restlessness, and, of course, sleeplessness. Caffeine is a diuretic, which means that it draws water out of body cells and tissues and increases the frequency of urination. Drinking caffeine after a certain time, say 6 P.M., can thus contribute to insomnia by making you get up and go to the bathroom in the middle of the night.

Caffeine also appears to inhibit the effects of both serotonin and another sleep-related neurotransmitter, melatonin, in the brain. Some evidence suggests that caffeine may act to reset the body's internal "clock." If so, then drinking caffeine late in the day may make your body think that it's morning again. It's hard to fall asleep when your body thinks it's seven in the morning.

Everyone knows that coffee is a major source of caffeine. (Even the decaffeinated variety retains a tiny amount.) But you may be surprised to know that caffeine is also an ingredient in a wide number of other products, including soft drinks, chocolate, coffee-flavored ice cream, hot cocoa, and most standard brands of tea (Table 4.2). If you are having trouble sleeping, you should first identify these sources of caffeine and eliminate them entirely from your diet.

Table 4.2: Caffeine Content of Common Beverages

Beverage	Caffeine (mg)
Coffee (7.5 oz. cup)	
Drip	115–150
Brewed	80–135
Instant	65–140
Decaffeinated	3–4
Tea (5 oz. cup)	
1-min. brew	20
3-min. brew	35
Iced (12 oz.)	70
Soft drinks	
Jolt	100
Mountain Dew	54
Tab	47
Coca-Cola	45
Diet Coke	45
Dr Pepper	40
Pepsi	38
Diet Pepsi	36
7Up	0

Different people have different sensitivity to caffeine, depending on how fast their metabolisms process the chemical and eliminate it from the body. That's why some people seem to be able to guzzle down potfuls of coffee and still drop off to sleep as soon as their head hits the pillow, while others can nibble a chocolate bar or sip a decaf latte and feel buzzed for hours.

Another substance that must be eliminated is alcohol. Although many people have a nightcap because they believe it will facilitate sleep, in fact alcohol can impair your ability to get a good night's rest. Alcohol triggers the release of adrenaline, one of your body's main natural stimulants.[5] What's more, alcohol impairs the transport of tryptophan into the brain, which in turn robs the brain of the raw material it needs to make serotonin.

Alcohol harms sleep by disrupting brain wave patterns and suppressing or delaying the REM phase. The presence of alcohol in the blood prevents the body from reaching the REM stage, especially during the first two or three ninety-minute sleep cycles. REM sleep is so important, however, that after your body metabolizes the alcohol, REM "rebound" occurs. This rebound involves more intense REM periods, as if your body is trying to make up for lost dream time. Several experts believe that drinking even small quantities of alcohol, less than one ounce, within an hour of bedtime can make your sleep light, unsettled, and unrefreshing.[6]

AVOID NOCTURNAL HYPOGLYCEMIA

In my clinical practice, I have found that nocturnal hypoglycemia (low nighttime blood glucose level) is an important cause of sleep-maintenance insomnia. When blood glucose levels drop, the body responds by releasing stimulating hormones such as adrenaline, glucagon, cortisol, and growth hormone, whose job, in part, is to regulate glucose levels. At the same time, though, these compounds stimulate the brain to send out strong signals telling your body that it is time for you to eat. Naturally, you can't sleep well if your body thinks its nutritional needs aren't being met. This, perhaps, is the biological basis for the time-honored tradition of the bedtime snack.

Many people in this country suffer from faulty glucose metabolism—either hypoglycemia or diabetes—because they eat too many refined carbohydrates, such as white sugar. If you like to nibble before turning in, choose snacks that will help you keep your blood sugar levels steady throughout the night. I recommend whole-grain breads or cereals, such as muffins or oatmeal. Besides controlling blood sugar levels, these complex carbohydrates promote sleep by increasing the level of the serotonin within the brain.

RELAX

Learn and practice techniques that promote relaxation and prepare the body and mind for sleep. One of the most popular and easy-to-use methods, progressive relaxation, works by helping you contrast the feeling of tension with that of relaxation. Once you are aware of the difference, you can learn to relax muscles one at a time until gradually your whole body is ready to drift away into restful slumber (see box below).

Relax . . . You Are Getting Sleepy . . .

Begin with the muscles in your face, such as those that move your eyebrows. Contract the muscles with gentle force for one to two seconds, and then relax. Don't stop breathing while you tense the muscles. Instead, you might want to count your breaths. Repeat a few times, then move on to the other muscles, such as those in the center of your face that control your nose and upper lip, and those that control the corners of your mouth.

Then tense and relax the muscles of the jaw and neck. Move on to the upper arms, the lower arms, and each finger of the hands. Eventually progress down the body, including the chest, the abdomen, the buttocks, the thighs, the calves, and finally the feet. Repeat the process two or three times.

In most cases, you won't be able to complete too many whole cycles, because you'll have relaxed yourself to sleep.

EXERCISE

People who regularly engage in exercise report fewer bouts of sleeplessness. Besides improving your general well-being, exercise promotes improved sleep quality by allowing smoother and more regular transition between the cycles and phases of sleep.

If possible, however, avoid exercise in the late evening or just before going to bed. Not surprisingly, exercise is stimulating to the body. It can take quite a while for your muscles and circulation system to calm down again after a vigorous workout.

Moderately intense exercise is all you need to enhance your ability to sleep well. Usually it is sufficient to get twenty minutes of aerobic exercise at a heart rate that is between 60 to 75 percent of maximum. (To calculate a good target heart rate range during exercise, subtract your age in years from 185 to determine the upper limit and subtract another 20 to determine the lower limit.)

If you try these lifestyle methods for a while—two to four weeks—and find you still aren't sleeping as well as you should, it may be time to move on to another approach. As I'll explain, 5-HTP can dramatically improve sleep quality and help you awake refreshed and ready to face the day.

5-HTP and the Treatment of Insomnia

Until the problem of contaminated L-tryptophan developed in the late 1980s, many people were taking doses of L-tryptophan as a strategy for dealing with insomnia. The logic was sound: L-tryptophan not only boosts serotonin levels, it also enhances the brain's ability to produce melatonin, the hormone that regulates your body's natural inner clock.[7] L-tryptophan also appears to reduce sleep latency (the time it takes you to fall asleep).[8]

As good as it was, though, L-tryptophan has *not* turned out to be an ideal natural method of promoting sleep. Clinical studies show that L-tryptophan produces only modest effects in the treatment of insomnia.[9] Not everyone who takes it for this purpose experiences the results they seek. People have to take relatively high doses of the substance (doses less than 2,000 mg are generally not effective).[10] More important, research shows that L-tryptophan can reduce REM sleep while increasing the time spent in non-REM sleep.[11]

Overall, 5-HTP is turning out to be a much more effective alternative for dealing with sleep problems in a safe and natural way. Several clinical studies show that 5-HTP produces dramatically better results than L-tryptophan in promoting and maintaining sleep in normal subjects as well as those experiencing insomnia.[12] According to these reports, the advantage of 5-HTP lies in its ability to improve sleep quality by increasing the length of time spent in both REM sleep and in deep sleep stages 3 and 4—*without increasing total sleep time.* 5-HTP accomplishes this by shortening the amount of time you spend in sleep stages 1 and 2, which in certain ways are the least important stages of the cycle.

These effects were first reported during the early 1970s in studies by Dr. Richard J. Wyatt at the National Institutes of Health in Bethesda, Maryland, and Dr. Vincent Zarcone at Stanford University. In the studies, subjects who received 200 mg of 5-HTP increased the amount of REM sleep by a total of about sixteen minutes over the five-day study. Those subjects taking 600 mg of 5-HTP increased total REM sleep time by an average of twenty minutes over five days. These results indicate that 5-HTP increases the amount of dream time by about three to four minutes a night—a small but significant amount. The higher the dose, the more time spent in REM.

By shifting the balance of the sleep cycle, 5-HTP makes sleep more restful and rejuvenating. Instead of waking feeling tired, worn out, and "hungover," people taking 5-HTP feel vibrant, well rested, and ready to take on the challenges of the day. When we sleep more deeply and dream more efficiently, we wake in the morning with our physical and psychological batteries fully charged.

The impact of 5-HTP on sleep stages is dose-related; taking higher doses produces a somewhat greater impact. In my clinical experience, however, the lower dosage is very adequate in most cases. Some patients who went against my advice and took higher doses reported that they experienced a greater number of disturbing dreams and nightmares. I attribute this risk to abnormally prolonged REM sleep. In addition, as I have discussed in the previous chapters, taking too much 5-HTP can lead to mild nausea.

To get the most out of the sleep- and dream-promoting effects of 5-HTP, I generally recommend taking 100 to 300 mg thirty to forty-five minutes before retiring. Start with the lower dose for at least three days, then consider increasing the dose if results are not what you expected. For added benefits, you might think about taking doses of passionflower, a natural herbal sleep enhancer that can add to the effects of 5-HTP. For more information, see Chapter 7.

5-HTP is quite remarkable in its ability to promote optimal sleep and dreaming, effects that in turn lead to greater mental, emotional, and physical rejuvenation. To illustrate, let me share the experience of one of my patients, Patty.

Java Jive:

PATTY'S STORY

Patty came to see me in April 1994 seeking relief for anxiety and insomnia. From her puffy, red eyes, I could tell right away that she was horribly sleep-deprived. During our initial conversation I learned that Patty, an attractive thirty-nine-year-old computer consultant, was going through some major life changes. When I reviewed my notes after our session, I remember thinking, "No wonder this woman can't sleep! What she's going through would keep anyone awake."

The stress level in Patty's life was off the charts. She was in the last stages of a difficult divorce from an abusive husband. Her attempts to date and to begin a new relationship were frustrating and unsuccessful. She had recently resigned from a full-time job and was trying to develop her freelance consulting business. At the same time she was hunting for a new apartment.

One of the biggest factors contributing to Patty's distress was her poor diet. Like many people living in Seattle, Patty had developed a great fondness for Starbucks coffee. She regularly consumed four "tall lattes" a day. If she wasn't drinking coffee, she could usually be spotted with a can of Diet Pepsi in her hand. I asked Patty if she ate breakfast. "Rarely," she replied, telling me that most of the time she opted instead for a double latte that she grabbed on her way to work. Her first solid "food" of the day was usually a midmorning Hershey bar from the vending machine. Lunch, her only significant meal of the day, was her saving grace: She often filled a plate from a salad bar, but on some days she settled for a fast-food sandwich and a bag of chips. For dinner at the end of her twelve-hour workdays, she usually had just a bowl of popcorn washed down with (you guessed it) a can of Diet Pepsi or another shot of java.

Patty told me she felt as though she was going nuts. "I just can't take it anymore," she said. Yes, she had been to other doctors and had tried a prescription drug (a benzodiazepine) for anxiety. She had also tried zolpidem (Ambien), a drug that is not a benzodiazepine (it's classified as a hypnotic of the imidazopyridine class) but which is often prescribed for insomnia. But she did not like the way these drugs made her feel. She complained of dizziness throughout the day and was especially unhappy with the diarrhea she attributed to these drugs. She had also tried, and had reacted quite negatively to, Prozac. "It jazzed me up so much I could hardly steer my car straight," she said. "And the fact that it made me lose my appetite for sex wasn't doing much for any budding romantic relationships."

She had come to me, she stated, in the belief that a more natural approach to treating her anxiety and insomnia represented her last resort. (I admit, I long for the day when more people will consider alternative treatments as their first resort.)

In my years of experience with patients, I have found that most people already know what they need to do to start solving their own problems. Often when they come to see me, what they are really seeking is an outsider, someone they perceive to be an expert, who will articulate and confirm their own inner feelings for them. With that in mind, I asked Patty what changes in her diet and lifestyle she thought she would need to make to improve the healthy functioning of her body and mind. "I need to eat better, cut down on caffeine, get some exercise," she said. "A perfect score," I replied.

I told Patty that much of the anxiety she was feeling resulted in large part from the changes going on in her life. She was faced with so many new situations that her body had kicked into fight-or-flight overdrive. For a body in such an agitated state, healthy, refreshing sleep is next to impossible. Yes, the divorce and the career moves and the hunt for new living space were all stressful. But seen in the proper light, with the right attitude, these could be considered as "good" stress—what some people call "eu-stress"—because they represented new opportunities, new goals, and positive new directions. "Right now," I told her, "your life is a big buffet of endless possibilities—enough to make anyone anxious. If you can taper off caffeine and get yourself sleeping right again, perhaps everything else will start falling into place. We need to find ways for you to transform the anxiety you feel into a healthier feeling of excitement—anxiety minus the fear."

I asked Patty some questions designed to get her thinking in this new direction. "What are the things in life that you are most excited about? Why does this make you feel excited?" As she answered those questions, I saw the first signs of an amazing transformation occur before my eyes. She saw that she could interpret her feelings in a new and more positive way, replacing anxiety and fear with excitement and hope.

I could sense that Patty was going to be okay. Still, I knew there were some steps we should take to get her body function back to normal so that her new, natural, positive mental attitude could take root and blossom.

I told her she had to cut out the candy bars and soft drinks. If she just couldn't let go of her beloved lattes, then at least switch to the decaf variety. I urged her never to skip breakfast, even if all she had was a piece of fruit and some orange juice, and to stick with salads at lunch. Popcorn is fine as a snack, but it's a lousy entree. I knew Patty would never find time or energy to cook dinner for herself, so I recommended some of the better microwaveable meals available from the grocery store, including vegetarian lasagna and some tasty bean casseroles. I also recommended membership in an exercise facility not far from where she was doing some apartment hunting. I suggested a high-potency multiple vitamin and mineral supplement. I also recommended a product containing kava extract. Kava (*Piper methysticum*) is a member of the pepper family native to the South Pacific. Based on the results of pharmacological and clinical studies, several European countries have approved kava preparations for the treatment of nervous anxiety, insomnia, and restlessness. I utilize kava extracts (standardized for kavalactone content) primarily in the treatment of anxiety and panic disorders. For this purpose, a typical regimen is 45 to 70 mg of kavalactones three times daily. As a sedative, the dosage of kavalactones is 80 to 210 mg, taken one hour before retiring. To promote sleep, I recommended taking 5-HTP a little before bedtime, starting with 100 mg and boosting it to 200 mg or 300 mg after a week or so if necessary.

Patty came back four weeks later. The difference was phenomenal. Her whole life had been transformed.

The first week had been tough, she admitted. Cutting out caffeine had triggered some pretty fierce withdrawal symptoms, including pounding headaches. (Acetaminophen helped, she said.) But after clearing that initial hurdle, she noticed that her energy levels were much higher. She felt "the weight of the world" had finally been lifted from her shoulders. For the first time in years she was sleeping like a baby. She was about to sign a lease for an apartment she loved. The divorce had been finalized. "And I'm having a blast flirting with the guy at the gym who uses the Stairmaster next to mine," she added with a smile.

Another comment she made caught my attention: Patty said she had started dreaming again. At the time I was treating Patty, my understanding of the role of 5-HTP in dreams was still somewhat limited. I assumed that the change in Patty's dreaming pattern resulted from her lower caffeine intake, or perhaps to the vitamin B_6, magnesium, or kava extract in her supplemental regimen.

Because Patty had managed to kick the caffeine habit, I suggested that she discontinue the 5-HTP. Two weeks later, though, she called to report that things were fine except that she "missed the dreams." And somehow her moods just weren't quite as elevated as they had been in the first four months of treatment. She asked if it would be a problem if she kept taking the 5-HTP. "Not at all," I replied, recommending a dose of 100 mg at bedtime.

I asked Patty to check in with me in a month. By that point Patty was doing great. Her dreams had returned, and so had her zest for living. This was two years ago. I asked her to check in with me every six months, and at each report she confirms that her sleep is sound and her life is on track.

5-HTP vs. Melatonin in Treating Insomnia

Melatonin has been called the body's own natural sleeping pill. It plays an important role in the sleep cycle by helping you fall asleep. Low melatonin levels can be a cause of sleep-onset insomnia. Since melatonin burst into the public consciousness a few years ago, millions of people have started taking this hormone to promote a good night's sleep.

The body's melatonin system works in an interesting way. First, the body changes serotonin into melatonin. Melatonin is then stored in the pineal gland inside the brain. The gland releases melatonin only during times when the level of light is low. Practically speaking, this means melatonin is secreted only at night, while you are asleep. In the morning, when you open your eyes, the presence of light is a sign to your brain to shut down the melatonin factory.

Several double-blind trials have shown that melatonin supplementation can be very effective in promoting sleep.[13] The hormone is most effective in people who have abnormally low levels of melatonin.[14] This is especially true in the elderly, because the efficiency of the melatonin system tends to decline with age.[15] If you have normal or high levels of melatonin, then taking a melatonin supplement will not result in increased sedation.

When you take 5-HTP, however, you bypass the brain's light-regulation system. 5-HTP leads to increased production of neurotransmitters, including serotonin and norepinephrine. High levels of these neurotransmitters in turn stimulate the noradrenergic receptors in the brain. This stimulation directly triggers the production and release of melatonin.[16] In short, taking 5-HTP causes melatonin release regardless of how much light is present.

With higher levels of melatonin in circulation, you are better able to fall asleep and stay asleep. People with low melatonin who take 5-HTP at nighttime will enjoy the same sedative effect as they will from taking melatonin alone, but they will also be getting the broader spectrum of benefits that comes from increased serotonin levels. In contrast, taking melatonin alone does not enhance these other important functions of the serotonin system. In a sense, the difference between taking melatonin and 5-HTP is the difference between taking a tablet containing a single vitamin and a tablet containing a few dozen crucial vitamins and minerals.

The effects of 5-HTP on melatonin depend on how much of the substance you take and at what time of day you take it. To produce enough neurotransmitter to override the brain's "light shutoff valve" that operates during the day, you would need to take relatively high doses of 5-HTP—more than 300 mg at a time. But unless you are trying to induce sleep during the daytime—for example, if you are trying to adjust to working on the night shift—you don't need to take this much 5-HTP.

The goal instead is to achieve normal nighttime sleep by making sure your body has stored up enough melatonin and to promote its release at night. The typical regimen I use in my practice to treat depression and insomnia (for example, 100 mg to 200 mg three times a day) promotes sleep as well. Taking 5-HTP at these doses helps your brain manufacture serotonin, some of which is then converted into melatonin and stored in the pineal gland. At bedtime, having adequate supplies of serotonin in the brain stimulates the release of melatonin—a process that is already under way due to the absence of light. Thus, taking standard doses of 5-HTP should enhance the body's own natural cycle of melatonin production and release without causing daytime sleepiness.

If you suffer from insomnia but not depression, then I recommend taking a single dose of 5-HTP at night. Start with a dose of 100 mg; if after a few days you don't see the results you want, increase the dose to 200 mg. In some cases, a single nighttime dose of 300 mg may be necessary. If depression is also a problem, then I recommend taking 100 to 200 mg of 5-HTP three times a day with meals. Some people do better if they take that third dose about forty-five minutes before bedtime.

I have recommended to many of my patients that they try switching from melatonin to 5-HTP as their nighttime sedative, and they all report better results with 5-HTP. They have an easier time falling asleep and staying asleep, enjoy healthy and memorable dream periods, and wake up without the morning grogginess that some patients experience with melatonin.

Sleepy Susan

Susan is a lively seventy-five-year-old woman, a former elementary school teacher and now a hospital volunteer (and one hell of a canasta player). As is typical for older individuals, Susan was having trouble sleeping at night.

"I just can't drop off the way I could before," she told me. She would lie on the bed trying to think calming thoughts, but her body just wouldn't cooperate. "After thrashing around for an hour I get up and fix a snack and try to read or watch TV or play solitaire. Gradually I get sleepy enough and doze off, sometimes right there in my easy chair. I wake up okay, but by midmorning I'm sleepy again. It's gotten so bad that now I'm liable to fall asleep whenever I'm sitting down. I can't get through a TV program or a *Reader's Digest* article before I start nodding off." Her insomnia was making it hard for her to complete her volunteer tasks at the hospital. "I hate it," she said. "I don't like sleeping while the sun is up and there are lots of things to do." Clearly, for Susan, her sleep patterns were interfering with her normal quality of life.

When I first started treating Susan, in late 1993, I suggested she try melatonin, a total dose of 3 mg, about half an hour before bedtime. At first she thought the treatment was working, but after a few weeks her insomnia was back. About this time I had begun to notice excellent improvement in the sleep habits of many of my patients who were taking 5-HTP for other purposes. I recommended that Susan try taking 5-HTP (300 mg at bedtime) instead of the melatonin.

Susan was delighted with the outcome. "Now I'm sleeping when I want to," she told me a few weeks later. Since she was getting her full rest during the night, she no longer felt as sleepy during the day. Knowing that she can enjoy her favorite activities again—reading, watching TV, volunteer work—has made a world of difference to her.

5-HTP and Treatment of Other Sleep Disorders

OBSTRUCTIVE SLEEP APNEA

The word *apnea* means "without breath." People with sleep apnea stop breathing for short periods of time—from ten to ninety seconds—while they are sleeping. During an episode, the brain sends strong signals to the body to make an all-out effort to start breathing again. The chest muscles heave and the lungs work hard to draw in air, usually accompanied by gasps and loud snorts. The sleeper rouses just enough to shift position. While normal people might experience four or five of these breathing-related arousals during the night, people with apnea have dozens, even hundreds, of apnea episodes every night.

Sleep apnea is not the same as snoring. When you snore, the air you inhale is being forced to pass through partially blocked passages (such as the nostrils or the back of the throat). But at least the air is moving. In sleep apnea, the air flow stops entirely until the body "jump-starts" itself, usually with a massive shudder and a loud snort.

Apnea severely interferes with sleep. During the episode, the person is aroused just long enough to start breathing again, but not usually long enough to remember being awake. In the morning, people with sleep apnea feel extremely groggy and unrested—and they have no idea why. They drag themselves through the day feeling sleepy and fatigued. The longer the condition persists, the more sleep-deprived they become. I discussed the deadly complications of sleep deprivation at the beginning of this chapter.

There are two primary types of sleep apnea. The more common type is called *obstructive sleep apnea,* or OSA. As the name indicates, OSA involves some kind of obstruction in the airway. It is more common among men than women, affecting one out of a hundred men between the ages of forty and seventy. Men who are overweight, even by just a few pounds, are especially susceptible. Other causes of OSA include hypothyroidism, enlarged tonsils, or narrowing of the nasal and respiratory passages due to chronic allergies or a birth defect.

The less common form of the condition, known as *central sleep apnea,* involves a problem in the nerve pathways that stimulate and control breathing. As a result, people with central sleep apnea may cease to breathe for periods of a few seconds, or their breathing may be too shallow or infrequent to provide sufficient oxygen to blood and tissues.

Decreased serotonin levels have been identified as one factor involved in sleep apnea.[17] The nerves that control breathing require an adequate supply of serotonin. Also, serotonin receptors control the release of hormones such as cortisol. One role of cortisol is to help control the muscles needed for breathing. Inspired by these findings, scientists have explored the question of whether serotonin-active substances produce improvements in apnea.

Many patients with OSA require assisted breathing at night using a device that delivers continuous positive airway pressure (CPAP). However, drug therapy can also help. Until recently, a tricyclic antidepressant, protriptyline, was the standard drug for treating OSA. As you have learned elsewhere in this book, the tricyclics block reuptake of both serotonin and norepinephrine. However, protriptyline causes such unpleasant side effects, including dry mouth, that many people quit taking the drug. Lately, the selective serotonin reuptake inhibitor Prozac has been used in treating OSA.[18] Prozac is equally effective but causes fewer side effects. A study in the early 1980s showed that L-tryptophan, a serotonin precursor, combined with protriptyline produced improvements in patients with OSA.[19] More recently, research conducted by Dr. D. A. Hanzel and colleagues at Case Western Reserve University in Cleveland has provided more evidence that the disturbed breathing in sleep apnea is a result of a malfunction in the serotonin system.[20] They conclude that, for at least some patients, the use of serotonin precursors such as 5-HTP may be of value.[21]

I have treated several patients with sleep apnea using 5-HTP as part of their overall medical care and have seen good results. My usual recommendation is 100 to 300 mg taken at bedtime. My patients report that they sleep more soundly and have fewer nighttime awakenings, which in turn helps them be more alert and productive during the day.

We need more studies to determine exactly which patients are most likely to benefit from 5-HTP and in what amounts. But so far the indications are that improving serotonin levels can help naturally restore healthy nighttime breathing patterns and reduce the suffering of apnea.

NARCOLEPSY

People with narcolepsy experience sudden, overpowering attacks of sleepiness lasting from a few seconds to half an hour. They might suffer dozens or even hundreds of these attacks each day. The attacks may be triggered by excitement or other intense emotions. Sleep lab studies show that narcolepsy results from a severe disturbance in the normal architecture of sleep. Specifically, people with narcolepsy go into the REM stage first, instead of at the end of a sleep cycle. Some evidence exists to suggest that taking 5-HTP may help some people with narcolepsy. In one study, a dose of 600 mg was found to have no effect on the number of sleep attacks. However, it did decrease the amount of time people with the disorder spent asleep during a daytime attack. What's more, it also lengthened the amount of time they slept at night.[22] More research is needed to define the possible role of 5-HTP in the treatment of narcolepsy.

PARASOMNIAS

Parasomnias are a group of sleep-related problems that includes grinding of the teeth (bruxism), night terrors, nightmares, sleepwalking, and talking while asleep. (Night terrors are sudden, intense episodes of fear and agitation that cause sudden awaken-

ing. These episodes occur during non-REM sleep, while nightmares are dreams that arise during the REM periods.)
Parasomnias can affect children as well as adults.

Research suggests that 5-HTP improves sleep quality in children and results in a lower incidence of nighttime awakenings,
night terrors, and other parasomnias.[23] The dosage of 5-HTP for
children is based on the child's weight: 4.5 mg per kilogram (2.2
pounds) per day. Remember to consult your child's pediatrician
before giving 5-HTP.

In adults, sleepwalking and other parasomnias usually result
from emotional stress. The most common parasomnia is restless
legs syndrome, which usually also involves nocturnal myoclonus.
Restless legs syndrome occurs when people are awake and involves an irresistible urge to keep moving the legs, either through
constant fidgeting or by walking around. Almost all patients with
restless legs syndrome also experience nocturnal myoclonus, a
condition that causes repeated muscular contractions of the legs
while sleeping. Most people with myoclonus don't know they have
the problem until they get complaints from their bed partner.
Many a mate has awakened with black-and-blue marks from being
kicked in the middle of the night by a myoclonus sufferer. The
condition also causes extreme daytime sleepiness. Some evidence
suggests that low serotonin levels may be a factor in this condition.

A recent study confirmed that iron deficiency in the blood can
contribute to restless legs syndrome, especially in the elderly.[24] A
blood test that measures levels of a protein called ferritin reveals
this iron shortage. Treatment with iron supplements can produce
good results. Many people also improve by boosting their levels of
the B vitamin called folic acid.

If your iron levels are normal, then 5-HTP may significantly
improve, or even eliminate, restless legs and myoclonus. A reasonable regimen calls for taking 100 to 200 mg of 5-HTP about
twenty minutes before retiring. However, do not take 5-HTP for
restless legs until you have had your iron levels checked, since

5-HTP will not supply you with iron your blood and your muscles need.

Treatment Recommendations for Sleep Disorders

The best approach to treating sleep problems is to identify and address the underlying cause. Common sense plays a big role here. Reducing stress and eliminating stimulants such as caffeine are usually the first steps. Getting exercise conditions the body and keeps its natural rhythms (including the sleep-wake cycle) operating at peak efficiency. The use of 5-HTP (or any other natural medicine, including melatonin) should begin only after nonpharmacologic treatments have proved ineffective. Once started, however, treatment with these natural medicines can be continued as long as necessary to restore and preserve sound, restful sleep.

For insomnia:
- Identify and address cause
- Eliminate caffeine and other compounds that interfere with sleep
- Try progressive relaxation techniques at bedtime
- Exercise
- 5-HTP: 100 to 300 mg at bedtime
- If you have insomnia and depression, take 100 to 200 mg three times a day and take the last dose forty-five minutes before retiring

Sleep apnea:
- Consult a physician for a complete evaluation of cardiovascular health

- Achieve ideal body weight
- Avoid alcohol consumption, especially within two hours before bedtime
- Use oxygen therapy if appropriate
- Consider surgery if above measures prove ineffective
- 5-HTP: 100 to 300 mg at bedtime

Parasomnias in Children:
- Rule out negative psychological stimuli (such as scary images from TV or books)
- 5-HTP: 4.5 mg per 2.2 pounds body weight

Parasomnias in Adults:
- Rule out negative psychological stimuli
- Rule out low iron levels
- 5-HTP: 100 to 300 mg at bedtime

Key Points of This Chapter

- Sleep disorders affect millions of Americans.
- Normal sleep is divided into two major phases: non-REM sleep and REM sleep (dream stage).
- Sleep cycles typically last up to ninety minutes and consist of a cycle of progressive non-REM sleep (stages 1–4) followed by episodes of REM sleep.
- Dreams are important for our daily physical and psychological renewal.
- About one person in three suffers from insomnia.
- The two main types of insomnia are sleep-onset insomnia

(trouble falling asleep) and sleep-maintenance insomnia (trouble staying asleep).

- The most common causes of insomnia are psychological: depression, anxiety, and tension.
- Medical conditions such as heart disease or chronic headaches can also trigger sleep disorder.
- Sleep problems are a potential side effect of over three hundred prescription medications.
- Poor diet, lack of exercise, and caffeine can contribute to low-quality sleep.
- Effective treatment of insomnia involves identifying and eliminating factors that disrupt sleep.
- The two major categories of sleeping pills are over-the-counter (antihistamines) and prescription (benzodiazepines and other kinds).
- Sleeping pills interfere with normal sleep patterns by affecting the amount of time spent in stage 3 and 4 sleep (deep sleep) and REM sleep.
- 5-HTP enhances REM sleep.
- The dosage for 5-HTP in insomnia is 100 to 300 mg thirty to forty-five minutes before retiring. Start with the lower dose for at least three days before increasing the dose.
- 5-HTP raises serotonin levels, and your body converts serotonin to melatonin. Serotonin also regulates the release of melatonin from the pineal gland during the night. For these reasons, 5-HTP can be a more effective sleep aid than melatonin.
- Low serotonin levels have been implicated in sleep apnea, and 5-HTP can boost serotonin levels to reduce apnea episodes and improve overall sleep quality.

- 5-HTP can help with parasomnias in children and adults.
- Do not stop taking or adjust dosages of any prescribed medication without first consulting your physician.
- If you snore at night, experience frequent nighttime wakenings, or feel tired and unrested during the day, see your physician for a medical evaluation.

CHAPTER 5

5-HTP AND HEADACHES

If you've read any of the previous chapters in this book, you can already predict why 5-HTP works so well against headaches. It corrects the biochemical defect that is the underlying cause of headache pain—low serotonin levels—and does so without causing the side effects associated with other medications. It also enhances the body's own pain-relief system, because serotonin controls the manufacture and release of beta-endorphins, which block pain signals in the nerves.[1]

Fortunately, most headaches are not serious threats to general health and well-being. Still, they are at the very least painful and annoying, and they certainly interfere with the enjoyment of daily living. In rare cases, headaches can arise from a major underlying illness, such as cancer or a brain tumor. Anyone with chronic recurring headaches should consult a doctor and have a complete medical evaluation.

There are basically two types of headaches. *Vascular* headaches are those that result from changes in blood vessels and cause throbbing or sharp, pounding pain. The pounding comes from blood pumping through veins and arteries with each beat of the heart. Migraines are a form of vascular headache. As you'll learn in this chapter, serotonin acts to constrict blood vessels and relieve pain. 5-HTP's effects on serotonin thus make it a valuable strategy for preventing headaches of this type.

In *nonvascular* headaches, the pain is steady and constant, ranging in severity from dull to excruciating. Usually the pain starts at the back of the head or in the forehead and spreads over the entire head. Many people who suffer from nonvascular headaches feel as though their head is caught in a vise and that an unseen hand is slowly ratcheting up the pressure. At this time, 5-HTP has not been shown to be of value in treating nonvascular headaches. There may be other indirect effects of 5-HTP on headache pain, such as improved mood or improved sleep, but as a rule I do not prescribe the product specifically for the treatment of headaches other than migraines.

Contrary to what many people believe, a headache is not a "pain in the brain." Brain tissue lacks sensory nerves. Instead, the pain arises within the three-layered membrane, called the meninges, that surrounds, protects, and nourishes the brain. Pain can also emanate from the scalp and its network of blood vessels and muscles.

Migraine headaches are caused by excessive dilation (expansion) of blood vessels in the head. Migraines are a surprisingly common disorder, affecting up to one person in every ten. These headaches occur three times more frequently among women. One reason for this is that women have higher levels of estrogen, and estrogen acts on blood vessels and increases blood pressure. In most cases, migraines first appear before age twenty; they can arise even in young children, often around age ten. Rarely do they emerge after age fifty. For more than half of migraine sufferers, there is evidence of a genetic susceptibility, since the condition tends to run in families. According to the National Headache Foundation, when both parents suffer from migraines, there is a 75 percent chance that a child will also have them. If one parent experiences migraines, there is a 50 percent chance that the child will get migraines.

Although many migraines strike without warning, migraine sufferers often experience a characteristic warning sign, called an aura, that appears before the onset of pain. Typically, an aura lasts a few minutes and causes blurring or bright spots in the vision, anxiety, fatigue, disturbed thinking, and numbness or tingling, usually on just one side of the body.

The most common nonvascular headache, called a tension headache, is caused by a tightening in the muscles of the face, neck, or scalp. Usually the tension results from stress or poor posture. As the muscles tighten, they pinch nearby nerves or blood vessels, triggering sensations of pain and pressure. Relaxing the muscle can bring about immediate relief. That's why so many people rub their temples during a tension headache—this spontaneous act eases the muscle spasm.

Overview of Headaches

Here are some pretty grim statistics to consider:

- Over forty-five million Americans get chronic, recurring headaches.
- Of these, sixteen to eighteen million people each year—70 percent of them women—get migraines.
- For some twelve million Americans, headaches occur every day.
- Industry loses $50 billion per year due to absenteeism and medical expenses caused by headache.
- Migraine sufferers lose more than 157 million workdays each year.
- Each year nearly fifty million people consult a doctor for help in dealing with headaches.
- Nearly 70 percent of adults in the United States take painkillers for a headache at least once a month.

- Americans spend more than $4 billion annually on over-the-counter pain relievers for headache, many of which are ineffective. *Some drugs even cause the very headaches they purport to relieve.*

For all chronic migraine headache sufferers, I have an important message: Give 5-HTP a try. It works.

Several clinical studies by Dr. N. T. Mathew of the Houston Headache Clinic have reported a shocking finding: Approximately seven out of ten people with chronic daily headaches experience pain caused directly by misuse of the very drugs they are taking in the hope of getting relief.[2] When these patients stop using these medications in excess (for example, when they stop taking doses of drugs every day to prevent headache), their headaches usually go away or are significantly reduced in frequency and severity. As a bonus, after withdrawing from the drug, they notice great improvements in their sleep patterns and in their general sense of well-being, with less irritability, depression, and lethargy.

Such conclusions—that, for many people, the headache "cure" can cause the disease—stand in stark contrast to results from clinical studies on 5-HTP. According to researchers at the University of Milan's Pain Research and Treatment Unit, anywhere from 77.4 to 93.5 percent of people with chronic daily headaches get better when they take 5-HTP.[3] This study lasted two months, and results continued to improve the longer the patients took 5-HTP. The same cannot be said for many prescription and OTC headache remedies, drugs that may lose their effectiveness or that, paradoxically, may even trigger headaches.

Escaping the Misery of Migraine:

SARA'S STORY

For Sara, migraine headaches had become a horribly routine part of her life. The instant she opened her eyes in the morning, she knew whether the day was going to produce yet another in a seemingly endless series of what she called her "cranial crises."

The throbbing would begin in a precise location, usually in the temples or near the knob at the back of her head, where her skull is attached to her spine. Like the beat of a drum in a demonic parade, the pounding would grow more and more intense. Eventually pain engulfed her whole head. Waves of nausea swept through her gut. When the monster had caught her fully in its grip, Sara was totally unable to think coherent thoughts, let alone get out of bed—except to vomit. The only thing she could do was lie in a dark room, a cold cloth draped over her forehead, praying for the waves of pain to subside.

If she was lucky, the agony wouldn't last more than twenty-four hours. "It's like labor," she quipped, "only you don't get a baby as your reward."

Her family was helpless. There was nothing they could do at these times except tiptoe around and occasionally bring her a fresh wet rag to drape on her forehead or some ice chips to suck on. Migraines aren't contagious. Still, when Sara had one, everyone in the house suffered.

But no one suffered like Sara. "Let me tell you how bad it is," she remarked to me. "I look forward to puking, because I know that's a sign the pain will start to let up."

By the time Sara came to see me, she had tried a lot of remedies. She had even summoned the courage to learn how to give herself injections of an antimigraine drug. "Poking a needle into my thigh is nothing compared to the pain of a migraine," she said. "It's the difference between sticking myself with a rose thorn and having someone swing a pickax at my head." The drug did help. Unfortunately, it also caused Sara to feel a persistent and worrisome tightness in her chest. "It was as if the migraine went away but left me a souvenir so I wouldn't ever forget it," said Sara. "My head didn't hurt so much, but I got really scared that my heart was about to give out."

At that point I asked Sara if she had ever heard of 5-HTP.

The Role of Serotonin in Headache

Although in this book we have focused on the role of serotonin on the brain, to understand its impact on migraine we have to explore the body a little further. In the 1940s American scientists discovered a chemical attached to the tiny blood particles called platelets. They soon found that this powerful chemical controlled the expansion and contraction of the muscles that surround the blood vessels. Because of these effects, they named the chemical serotonin—*sero-* for "blood," *tonin* for "muscle tone."

As you learned in Chapter 1, there are various subgroups of serotonin receptors that serve different functions. Like the brain, the cells in the blood vessels also contain several types of serotonin receptors. When serotonin binds to one of these subtypes (known as $5-HT_{1D}$), blood vessels contract. (5-HT is short for 5-hydroxytryptamine, the chemical name for serotonin.) Another subtype, known as $5-HT_{1C}$, causes the vessels to widen (dilate) again.

Low levels of serotonin can cause these various receptors to become overly sensitive. To understand what I mean, think about what happens when you walk from outside on a sunny day into a dark room. Once you step inside, the pupils of your eyes start to expand as they adjust to the darkness. What's happening is that your eyes are trying to compensate for the lack of light. The pupils widen (or dilate) to become more sensitive, to pick up whatever light is available and thus help you to see better. Conversely, if you walk from a dark room into bright daylight, your pupils shrink again to prevent too much light from entering the eye.

In a sense, the same thing happens with serotonin receptors. Lack of serotonin causes the receptors to develop increased sensitivity to the neurotransmitter. Whereas normally it might take, say, ten molecules of serotonin to trigger a nerve impulse, in people with low serotonin levels the same impulse might require only one or two molecules of serotonin. In this way, the body is doing what it can to make up for the absence of serotonin—just as the widening pupils of your eye make up for the absence of light.

But this increased sensitivity comes with a price. As you know, walking from a dark room into bright sunlight can be painful. Similarly, when the serotonin receptors that control blood vessel dilation grow too sensitive, then the presence of even small quantities of serotonin can trigger sudden excessive widening of the vessels. When that happens, the blood flow through the vessels increases. This, in turn, leads to vascular complications—including the pounding throb of migraine. Of course, the receptors that constrict the vessels may also be more sensitive. But as it happens, the receptors governing dilation seem to be more powerful than those controlling constriction. In this biochemical tug-of-war, the dilation receptors win.[4]

The bottom line: Low serotonin levels can lead to painful headaches.[5]

There are a number of factors that can trigger the release of serotonin, not just from the neurons in the brain, but from the platelets in the blood. A list of these factors appears in Table 5.1. When serotonin enters the bloodstream of people who suffer from chronic low serotonin, the result can be a migraine. Conversely, raising serotonin levels back to normal decreases the sensitivity of the neurons and restores better, more balanced control over the blood vessels. That's why increasing serotonin by taking 5-HTP can control migraines.

Table 5.1: Factors That Trigger Headaches

- Low serotonin levels (possible genetic factor)
- Foods
    - Food allergies
    - Histamine-releasing foods
    - Histamine-containing foods
- Alcohol, especially red wine

- Chemicals
  - Monosodium glutamate (MSG)
  - Nitrates
  - Nitroglycerin
- Withdrawal from caffeine or other drugs that constrict blood vessels
- Stress
- Emotional changes, especially letdown after stress or intense emotions such as anger
- Hormonal changes (such as menstruation, ovulation, birth control pills)
- Too little or too much sleep
- Exhaustion
- Poor posture
- Muscle tension
- Weather changes (such as changes in barometric pressure, exposure to sun)
- Glare or eyestrain

Back in the 1960s researchers discovered that, during the course of a migraine, people produce higher levels of a substance called 5-HIAA.[6] As you may remember from earlier in this book, 5-HIAA (the short name for 5-hydroxyindoleacetic acid) is a substance that results when the body breaks down molecules of serotonin. This by-product gets washed out of the body in the urine. We know, then, that the higher the level of 5-HIAA in the urine, the more serotonin the body is making and releasing.

But wait a minute, you may be saying to yourself. If during a migraine our bodies produce *higher* levels of serotonin, then wouldn't that suggest that *increased* serotonin causes the migraine?

Good question. And initially that's what a lot of scientists thought. More recent research, however, shows that the opposite is true. We now know that during a migraine episode, our bodies do not necessarily produce more serotonin. Instead, what happens is that they are releasing the available supply of serotonin that has been stored in cells in a desperate effort to relieve the headache. Thus, during a migraine, more serotonin is present in the spaces between brain cells. When the serotonin level goes up, the enzyme called monoamine oxidase (MAO) kicks into high gear. The function of MAO is to break up serotonin as fast as it can.[7] The more MAO does its job, the higher the level of 5-HIAA that will show up in the urine.

Many of the prescription drugs available for migraine are designed to affect the serotonin system. Sumatriptan, sold under the brand name Imitrex, is classified as a serotonin *agonist*. The word *agonist* means that the drug enhances the effects of serotonin. (In contrast, an *antagonist* blocks the activity of another drug.) Imitrex activates the 5-HT_{1D} receptors and thus helps the blood vessels constrict. Imitrex is now among the most widely prescribed headache medications. Another major migraine drug, Sansert (methysergide), works in a different way. It blocks the 5-HT_{1C} receptors and thus prevents the blood vessels from dilating.

In addition, the antidepressants classified as monoamine oxidase inhibitors (MAOIs) are also sometimes prescribed for headache. These drugs block the activity of MAO, the enzyme that breaks down serotonin, and thus help preserve the supply of this valuable neurotransmitter.

Prescription drugs are effective, no doubt about it. But they can also cause serious side effects, as I'll explain in a moment. 5-HTP, however, provides the same benefits by boosting serotonin levels, reducing receptor sensitivity, and preventing migraines—and it does so without adverse effects.

The process of adjusting the basic level of sensitivity of 5-HT receptors is a gradual one. It may take time for the effects to be noticed. This fact explains why, in many cases, the benefits of 5-HTP for headache prevention increase over time. Studies show that people taking 5-HTP experience fewer headaches after sixty days of continuous treatment than they do at the thirty-day mark.[8]

As I have said, when brain serotonin levels are low, your perception of pain is heightened. One reason for this is that without enough serotonin present, your brain can't produce and release adequate levels of endorphins.[9] Endorphins are the body's natural opiate system, responsible for damping pain as well as elevating mood. Endorphins work exactly the same way in the body as narcotics such as opium and morphine. That is, all of these chemicals bind to the same receptors and block the perception of pain. Many scientists believe that the pain-relieving and mood-elevating benefits of 5-HTP may reflect 5-HTP's impact on endorphin levels rather than its direct effect on serotonin.

Whatever the case may be, one fact remains: 5-HTP can relieve the pain and suffering for millions of headache sufferers.

5-HTP vs. Other Headache Drugs and Treatments

Let's move from the biology lab out into the real world. The news here is very good: Several clinical studies on 5-HTP in the treatment of vascular headaches have produced excellent results. 5-HTP is especially valuable for preventing migraines, and it has a lower risk of significant side effects than prescription drugs (Table 5.2).

Table 5.2: Common Drugs for Preventing
Migraine Headaches

Drug	Adult Daily Dosage	Common Side Effects
Aspirin	650–1950 mg	Gastric irritation, ulcer formation
Calcium channel blockers—Calan (verapramil), Procardia (nifedipine), Cardizem (diltiazem), etc.	80–160 mg	Headache, low blood pressure, flushing, water retention, constipation
Catapres (clonidine)	0.2–0.6 mg	Dry mouth, drowsiness, sedation, headache, constipation
Elavil (amitriptyline); Tofranil (imipramine)	10–150 mg	Drowsiness, dry mouth, constipation, weight gain, blurred vision, water retention
Inderal (propranolol)	80–240 mg	Fatigue, lassitude, depression, insomnia, nausea, vomiting, constipation
Periactin (cyproheptadine)	12–20 mg	Sedation, dry mouth, gastrointestinal disturbances

Prozac (fluoxetine)	20–60 mg	Anxiety, insomnia, sweating, tremor, gastrointestinal disturbances
Sansert (methysergide)	4–8 mg	Nausea, vomiting, diarrhea, abdominal pain, cramps, weight gain, insomnia, edema, decreased blood flow to extremities, heart and lung fibrosis
Zoloft (sertraline)	50–200 mg	Anxiety, insomnia, sweating, tremor, gastrointestinal disturbances

Source: E. Sanders-Bush and S. E. Mayer, "5-hydroxytryptamine (serotonin) receptors and antagonists," in J. G. Hardman and L. E. Limbird, eds. *Goodman and Gilman's Pharmacological Basis of Therapeutics, Ninth Edition* (New York: McGraw-Hill, 1996).

The problem of prescription drug therapy for preventing migraine headaches is perhaps best illustrated by Sansert (methysergide). As I noted above, this commonly prescribed drug inhibits the serotonin receptor that can trigger a headache. Sansert is generally regarded as the most effective antimigraine drug available by prescription, showing results in 60 to 80 percent of cases. But side effects are common and can be severe. In August 1994 the FDA ordered Sansert's manufacturer, Sandoz, to put a "black box" warning label on the product. This warning alerts users to the fact that long-term use of Sansert can trigger a serious form of lung and heart disease called fibrosis. This condition causes thick, fibrous patches to develop in tissues, interfering with their ability to function. People taking the drug must notify their physicians immediately if they develop symptoms such as cold, numb, and painful hands and feet; painful leg cramps while walking; or pain of any type occurring in the abdomen or chest. These complications limit the use of the drug. Patients must stop taking it after six months and then wait for another three or four weeks before they can begin again.

Sansert and 5-HTP work in completely different ways. The prescription medication inhibits or blocks the effects of serotonin at the headache-causing receptors. In contrast, 5-HTP boosts serotonin levels, which over time desensitizes the headache-causing receptors while enhancing activity at the headache-preventing receptors. 5-HTP is not known to cause the adverse effects seen with methysergide, such as lung or heart fibrosis.

Clinical studies comparing the two treatments underscore the benefits of 5-HTP. In a large double-blind study in Barcelona at the Headache Unit of the Hospital Valle Hebron, 5-HTP was compared to methysergide (the active ingredient in Sansert) in patients suffering from frequent migraine headaches.[10] Patients received six months of treatment with either 5-HTP (600 mg daily) or methysergide (3 mg daily) for six months. Treatment was considered successful if the patient experienced a 50 percent or greater reduction in frequency or severity of attacks. In terms of outcome, results in the two groups were basically the same: 75 percent (30 out of 40 patients) taking methysergide and 71 percent (32 out of 45) of those taking 5-HTP improved or had no more attacks (Table 5.3). In scientific terms, these results are a statistical dead heat.

The real advantage of 5-HTP over the drug was in the incidence of side effects. Thirteen out of forty-five subjects (about 29 percent) taking 5-HTP at a dosage of 600 mg a day experienced nausea that was both mild and temporary. Five patients in the methysergide group dropped out of the study because of side effects, but no one taking 5-HTP dropped out. The authors concluded, "These results suggest that 5-HTP could be a treatment of choice in the prevention of migraine."

Table 5.3: 5-HTP vs. Methysergide for Headache

	Methysergide	5-HTP
No attacks (100% reduction)	35%	25%
Improvement (>50% reduction)	40%	46%
No improvement	12.5%	29%
Withdrawal due to side effects	12.5%	0%

Source: F. Titus et al., "5-Hydroxytryptophan versus methysergide in the prophylaxis of migraine: Randomized clinical trial," *European Neurology* 25 (1986): 327–29.

While these studies used a dosage of 600 mg daily, equally impressive results were achieved at doses as low as 200 mg daily in double-blind studies conducted by Federigo Sicuteri at the University of Florence in Italy.[11] In these trials, 70 percent of patients taking 5-HTP for two months experienced significant improvement—the same rate as seen with Sansert—but 5-HTP did not cause side effects. The bottom line is that 5-HTP is at least as effective as these standard drug treatments and is certainly much safer and better-tolerated.

In my practice, I have seen excellent results in many migraine patients even when they take low doses of 5-HTP. As a rule, it's always smart to take the lowest possible effective dose. If you are considering taking 5-HTP for migraine prevention, I recommend starting at a dosage of 50 mg three times per day. After two weeks, if you are not experiencing significant improvement, try increasing the dose to 100 mg three times per day. Stick with this regimen for at least two months (remember, it takes time for serotonin activity to alter the sensitivity of the receptors). If after that time you still experience headaches, increase the dosage to 150 mg four times per day (a dose taken at each meal and again at bedtime) to achieve a daily dose of 600 mg. Continue your treatment for as long as necessary to provide relief.

Laurie

Laurie is a twenty-two-year-old college student. During our first meeting, she pulled a family photo from her wallet and pointed out her mother. "We're a lot alike," she said. "We have the same eyes, the same hair, the same sense of humor—and the same lousy headaches."

Laurie had inherited the "family curse," as she put it—severe migraines that would strike from one to three times a week, rendering her miserable and incapacitated. She called her migraine episodes the "black holes" in her life. She had experienced her first migraine around the age of twelve, just about the time she had her first period. "The cramps and bloating aren't enough," she complained. "I have to endure having my head put through the wringer as well."

In their quest for relief over the years, both Laurie and her mother had tried a range of treatments, conventional as well as alternative. Some methods worked for a while, but eventually the treatment would lose its effectiveness or would cause worrisome side effects. She had heard about Imitrex, which at that time was available only as an injectable drug, but refused to try it because she hated the thought of giving herself regular injections. I suggested that Laurie try 5-HTP, 200 mg three times a day. I urged her to be patient, because it might take a few months for the full benefit to appear.

After three weeks Laurie reported that the migraines continued, but they seemed to be less severe and less frequent. At the two-month mark she called me, and the excitement in her voice was clear. She was just about headache-free. Meanwhile her mother had also started taking 5-HTP and was experiencing good results. Three months later I spoke to Laurie again; she had experienced only two headaches in that time and they had both been mild.

With 5-HTP, the "black holes" in Laurie's life had vanished.

5-HTP for Treating Children's Headaches

Many children suffer enormously from severe, recurring headaches, including migraines. One of the best potential uses of 5-HTP is in providing relief to these kids without the higher risk of side effects posed by prescription drug treatments. Several studies on 5-HTP in the treatment of chronic headaches in children and adolescents have produced excellent results.[12]

A study at the Institute of Children's Psychiatry at the University of Rome involved forty-eight elementary and junior high students suffering from recurrent headaches (at least one headache every two weeks). The students were divided into two groups. One group started by taking the placebo for two months and then switched to 5-HTP. (Dosage was based on the child's weight: 4.5 mg per kilogram, or 2.2 pounds. The dose was divided into two administrations per day.) The other group took 5-HTP for two months, after which the patients were supposed to be switched to placebo. However, nine of these children *refused to switch* because they were doing so well on the 5-HTP. Remember, too, that this was a blind study, in which the patients were not supposed to know whether they were getting the active substance. These kids knew, however. How? Simple. Their headaches had vanished. Because of this situation, in order to assess their data the study team had to divide some of the patients into a third group, made up of those who remained on 5-HTP and who did not switch over to the placebo.[13]

The researchers measured outcomes using a tool called the headache index. To calculate the index, the number of headaches occurring in one month is multiplied by the intensity of the headache (measured on a scale of 1 to 3). Using this headache index as their yardstick, the investigators found that headaches were reduced by about 70 percent when the kids were taking 5-HTP (Table 5.4). In contrast, the index fell by only 11.5 percent during the placebo phase. And it's no wonder those nine rebellious patients refused to give up their treatment; among this group, there was a whopping 81.8 percent decrease in the headache index after the second month. To underscore the importance of long-term treatment with 5-HTP for headaches, this same subgroup of highly responsive patients showed only an 18.2 percent reduction at the one-month mark.

Table 5.4: Headache Scores During Treatment with 5-HTP and Placebo (% Improvement on Headache Index Rating Scale)

Group	Protocol	1 mo.	2 mo.	3 mo.	4 mo.
A	5-HTP for 2 months, then placebo	18.0	71.5	85.0	82.0
B	Placebo for 2 months, then 5-HTP	−20.0*	15.0	55.0	69.6
C	5-HTP for 2 months	18.2	81.8	—	—

* Negative number indicates headaches grew worse during placebo treatment.

Source: G. De Giorgis et al., "Headache in association with sleep disorders in children: A psychodiagnostic evaluation and controlled clinical study: L-5-HTP versus placebo," *Drugs Under Experimental and Clinical Research* 13 (1987): 425–33.

One impressive aspect of this study is the fact that the benefits of 5-HTP occurred without side effects. Not a single child complained of adverse reactions while taking 5-HTP. For some reason, these children seemed to be less vulnerable to the mild nausea commonly associated with 5-HTP treatment. I have also found this to be true in my practice (although, for that matter, I do not hear many of my patients complain about even mild nausea with 5-HTP treatment).

The possible benefits of 5-HTP in children with recurrent headache are far-reaching. The forty-eight children in the De Giorgis trial were doing less well in school than their classmates. Their intellectual capacity was normal, but the combination of debilitating headaches, poor sleep, and possible depression was keeping them from succeeding in the classroom. As far as I know, taking 5-HTP won't increase a kid's IQ, but clearly if people sleep well, enjoy a normal mood, and are free from pounding pain in the head, they are more likely to stay alert and productive in school.

In my opinion, a trial of 5-HTP for two months in young people with chronic headaches certainly seems reasonable.

> **Always consult a pediatrician before giving 5-HTP to a child.**

Effects of 5-HTP on Beta-Endorphin Levels in Juvenile Headache

In addition to its impact on serotonin, 5-HTP may relieve headaches (both the vascular and nonvascular varieties) by affecting levels of beta-endorphins.[14]

A clinical trial at the Department of Pediatrics at the University of Padua in Italy studied the effects of 5-HTP in twenty juvenile patients who suffered from either migraines or tension headaches.[15] The researchers measured the patients' levels of both serotonin and beta-endorphins and compared those results to those from a group of young people who did not suffer from headaches.

Patients were monitored and evaluated for frequency and intensity of headache attacks for three months prior to 5-HTP treatment and during another three months of therapy. The total headache score was calculated by multiplying the frequency of attacks by their severity. Here is the scoring system used:

Frequency:

    0   No attack
    1   Less than 1 attack per month
    2   1–3 attacks per month
    3   More than 3 attacks per month

Severity:

0   No attack

1   Mild

2   Moderate

3   Severe

Results showed that 5-HTP produced a statistically significant reduction in the headache scores in both migraine and tension-type headache sufferers. Based on measurements of neurotransmitters, the researchers attributed the improvement primarily to increased beta-endorphin levels (Table 5.5). Even though 5-HTP raised the level of beta-endorphins, the levels were still much lower than those found in the control group of people who did not suffer from headaches. This suggests that young people may need to keep taking 5-HTP for long periods—up to six months or more—before they will experience an increase in beta-endorphins sufficient to provide headache relief.

Table 5.5: Effect of 5-HTP on Levels of Serotonin and Beta-Endorphins

	Serotonin (serum mcg/L)	Beta-Endorphin (plasma pmol/L)	Beta-Endorphin (white blood cells pmol/10^6 GB/L)
Migraine (13 subjects)			
Before	104.6	16.2	110.5
After	115.7	19.4	120.3
Tension-type (7 subjects)			
Before	90.7	14.5	142.3
After	97.2	17.6	152.4

Total (20
subjects)

Before	100.5	15.7	129.3
After	108.3	18.4	· 140.4
Controls (17 subjects)	96.0	21.3	359.3

These results may also indicate that 5-HTP alone may not raise beta-endorphin levels enough to relieve headache. Other therapies designed to increase beta-endorphin levels, including exercise, acupuncture, and biofeedback, can be used in combination with 5-HTP to enhance its effects.

Treatment Recommendations for Chronic or Recurring Headaches

Effective treatment for recurrent headaches first involves identifying and addressing the underlying cause. First, see a qualified medical professional to get a complete evaluation. There are many hospitals and treatment centers that offer workups specifically for headache.

Next, follow a healthy lifestyle, eat a nutritious diet, and use 5-HTP. I have also found that supplements, including magnesium and vitamin B_6, can provide additional benefits. (For more information, see Chapter 7.)

Dietary and Lifestyle Recommendations:
- Consume a whole-foods diet (whole grains, legumes, vegetables, fruits, nuts, and seeds)
- Eliminate alcohol, caffeine, and sugar
- Identify and control food allergies
- Get regular exercise
- Perform a relaxation exercise (deep breathing, meditation,

prayer, visualization, etc.) for ten to fifteen minutes each day
- Drink at least 48 ounces of water daily
- Cut out foods and drinks that contain histamine (such as chocolate, cheese, wine, and beer), since histamine can trigger migraine headaches

Supplement Protocol:
- 5-HTP: 100 to 200 mg three times daily
- Vitamin B$_6$: 25 to 50 mg three times daily
- Magnesium: 250 to 400 mg three times daily; organic forms of magnesium (citrate, malate, or aspartate) are absorbed better and tolerated better than inorganic forms (such as magnesium sulfate, hydroxide, or oxide), which tend to act as laxatives

Warning

People with severe kidney disease or severe heart disease (such as high-grade atrio-ventricular block) should not take magnesium or potassium unless under the direct advice of a physician.

Key Points of This Chapter

- Effective treatment for headache requires appropriate identification of the underlying and precipitating factor(s).
- Prescription drugs used to treat and prevent headaches are

associated with numerous and sometimes severe—even fatal—side effects.

- Paradoxically, continued use of headache medications can lead to chronic daily headache.
- Food allergy is a major cause of chronic headache.
- Foods such as red wine, chocolate, cheese, and aspartame can lead to histamine-induced headaches.
- 5-HTP has been proved effective in double-blind studies in patients with recurrent migraine headaches.
- Do not stop taking or adjust dosages of any prescribed medication without first consulting your physician.
- If you suffer from severe recurrent headaches, see your physician for a medical evaluation.
- Do not take magnesium or potassium supplements if you have kidney disease or heart disease.

CHAPTER 6

5-HTP AND FIBROMYALGIA, PMS, AND OTHER CONDITIONS

In addition to depression, obesity, insomnia, and headaches, there are several other conditions that cause enormous suffering to millions of people and that may also respond to treatment with 5-HTP. These include:

- Fibromyalgia
- Chronic fatigue syndrome
- Premenstrual syndrome
- Parkinson's disease
- Seizure disorders

Fibromyalgia

Many people come to see me because they are experiencing a tremendous sense of overall pain. I can't tell you how many times I've heard someone say, "I hurt all over," or "My muscles just ache all the time," or "I'm so tired but I can't seem to get a good night's sleep." Their pain is constant and gnawing, and it profoundly interferes with their ability to function at home or at work. Often these people have seen a series of doctors, but each time they have been told that their complaints and symptoms are too vague or general to be a "real" condition. When doctors can't pinpoint the problem, they often send patients out the door with a prescription for a pain reliever and the none-too-helpful suggestion that they "will just have to learn to live with it."

Fortunately, that situation is changing. In the past few decades medical science has grudgingly recognized that a general syndrome of pain, stiffness, and disturbed sleep does indeed exist. Its name: fibromyalgia.

— Oddly enough, the term *fibromyalgia* doesn't even appear in some current medical dictionaries. But it's a real condition, all right. The Greek roots of the word refer to pain in the muscles and connective tissues. Originally some researchers thought fibromyalgia might be a form of arthritis or joint disease. We now know, however, that the condition primarily affects the muscles. In past decades, the syndrome was often referred to as fibrositis or fibromyositis. The trouble with those names is that *-itis* indicates some form of inflammation. In fibromyalgia, however, the muscles are not inflamed, but they are stiff and painful.

The main symptom in fibromyalgia is an overall body pain, which in many cases leads to severe fatigue. A somewhat similar condition, chronic fatigue syndrome, causes overwhelming tiredness, and in many cases also involves general body pain. I discuss chronic fatigue syndrome later in this chapter.

Fibromyalgia is a common condition, affecting between 3 and 6 percent of the population in this country—as many as sixteen million people.[1] In most cases, fibromyalgia strikes people between the ages of twenty and sixty, but it can occur in both younger and older individuals. Three out of four sufferers are women. Despite the fact that fibromyalgia is so widespread, doctors often fail to make the diagnosis. As a result, many people suffer needlessly for years before they find a name for what ails them. Until the diagnosis is made, effective treatment cannot begin.

The disorder produces somewhat different patterns in different people (Table 6.1). In all cases, though, a generalized pain is involved, usually affecting the neck, shoulders, lower back, hips, shin, elbows, or knees. The pain is typically worse in the morning. Most patients also experience severely disturbed sleep. Not surprisingly the burden of chronic pain coupled with inadequate restorative sleep can contribute to depression.

Recognize the pattern? As we have seen in previous chapters, all of these chief complaints arising from fibromyalgia are associated with abnormally low levels of serotonin.

Table 6.1: Diagnostic Criteria for Fibromyalgia

For a diagnosis of fibromyalgia to be made, the patient must meet all three major criteria and four or more of the minor criteria:

- Major criteria
    - Generalized aches or stiffness in at least three anatomic sites for at least three months
    - Six or more typical, reproducible tender points
    - Exclusion of other disorders that can cause similar symptoms
- Minor criteria
    - Generalized fatigue
    - Chronic headache
    - Sleep disturbance
    - Neurological and psychological complaints
    - Joint swelling
    - Numbness or tingling sensations
    - Irritable bowel syndrome

• Variation of symptoms in relation to activity, stress, and weather changes

Source: Centers for Disease Control and Prevention.

In addition to overall aches and fatigue, fibromyalgia can cause headaches, memory and concentration problems, dizziness, numbness and tingling, general itchiness, fluid retention, cramps in the abdomen, pelvic pain and diarrhea, and perhaps other symptoms as well. Often people with the syndrome are sensitive to extremely warm or cold temperatures. Fibromyalgia can cause a reduced ability to tolerate exercise, even mild exercise such as walking. Fortunately, fibromyalgia is not a life-threatening condition, nor does it cause permanent deformity. However, it is a chronic (persistent, recurring, and long-term) problem. Although fibromyalgia can be managed, there is no known cure. In most cases, people with the syndrome will need to find ways of dealing with it for the rest of their lives.

It's not surprising that the diagnosis of fibromyalgia is so often missed. There is no diagnostic test or X ray that can detect the syndrome. However, as the major criteria in Table 6.1 show, fibromyalgia involves sensitivity to painful pressure at specific places in the body. These "fibromyalgia pressure points" are indicated in Figure 6.1.

Because 5-HTP improves sleep and relieves the sensation of pain, it can be a boon for people suffering from fibromyalgia. As is often the case in science, the discovery that serotonin may be involved in this condition arose by accident.

Back in the early 1970s Dr. Sicuteri at the University of Florence in Italy was searching for a treatment for migraine headache.[2] He was studying the role of serotonin in migraines. As you may remember from Chapter 5, for many years researchers mistakenly assumed that severe headaches resulted from *increased* levels of serotonin. That's because they had measured the urinary levels of 5-HIAA, the breakdown product that results when the body metabolizes serotonin. Because people with migraines pro-

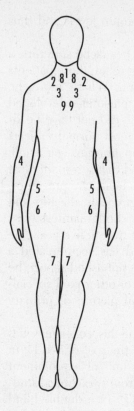

Location of FMS tender points:

1) Attachment of neck muscles at the base of the skull
2) Midway between neck and shoulder
3) Muscle over upper inner shoulder blade
4) 2 cm below side bone at elbow
5) Upper outer buttock
6) Hip bone
7) Just above knee on inside
8) Lower neck in front
9) Edge of upper breast bone

Figure 6.1: Fibromyalgia Pressure Points

duce very high levels of 5-HIAA during the headache episode, scientists believed that high serotonin must be the culprit. As it turns out, the body is actually releasing a flood of serotonin in a valiant effort to counteract the pain.

Meanwhile, back to our story. In his quest for a migraine cure, Dr. Sicuteri conducted studies on a drug called _fenclonine._ This agent works by interfering with the enzyme that converts molecules of tryptophan into molecules of 5-HTP. The more active this enzyme, the faster the body can produce 5-HTP—the raw material the brain needs to make serotonin. By slowing down the enzyme, the scientist hoped to reduce serotonin levels and thus relieve the agony of migraine.

But when Dr. Sicuteri gave fenclonine to headache sufferers, a surprising thing happened. Instead of getting relief, these patients began experiencing excruciating muscle pain. What's more, he found that people with migraines who took fenclonine developed much more severe pain than did people who did not have headaches. In fact, his experiments showed that most normal subjects who were given fenclonine did not develop fibromyalgia at all. With a flash of insight, the researcher realized that serotonin must be acting not as a headache inducer but as a headache preventer.

Dr. Sicuteri became convinced that migraine headaches and fibromyalgia share a common origin: They are both manifestations of a low-serotonin syndrome.[3] Over the past twenty-five years, he has treated many patients with 5-HTP and has accumulated a mountain of evidence to make his case. In a published report, he notes: "In our experience, as well as in that of other pain specialists, 5-HTP can largely improve the painful picture of primary fibromyalgia."[4]

The success reported by Dr. Sicuteri and his colleagues has inspired other Italian researchers to explore the role of 5-HTP in fibromyalgia. A group at the rheumatology unit of a prominent hospital in Milan reported excellent results from two clinical studies on treatment of fibromyalgia with 5-HTP. In a double-blind study, fifty patients were divided into two groups. The group that received 5-HTP (100 mg) per day showed significant improvement in their symptoms, while the placebo group experienced virtually no improvement.[5] Two patients in each group dropped out, leaving a total of forty-six in the final assessment.

As shown in Table 6.2, 5-HTP was rated significantly better than placebo both by the patients and by their evaluating physicians. Improvements were noted in all symptom categories: number of painful areas, morning stiffness, sleep patterns, anxiety, and fatigue. Intriguingly, although 5-HTP produces very good results within a short period of time, the improvement was even better after thirty days of treatment. Similarly, in the second study, patients who took 100 mg of 5-HTP three times daily reported maximum results at thirty days; benefits of the treatment continued at that level through the rest of the ninety-day trial.[6]

Table 6.2: Response to 5-HTP vs. Placebo in Fibromyalgia

Response	5-HTP	Placebo
Good	11	1
Fair	8	5
Poor	4	8
None	0	9

One of Dr. Sicuteri's larger studies involved 319 people with fibromyalgia.[7] After a month on placebo, 219 patients received L-tryptophan (2,000 mg daily) while the remaining 100 received 5-HTP (200–400 mg daily) for one year. Either treatment led to significant improvements in muscle pain and sleep disturbance. However, the researchers studied the data further by grouping the patients according to age (nine to eighteen years, twenty to thirty-seven, and thirty-eight to fifty-eight). They found an interesting pattern: The younger group enjoyed the greatest improvement, while the older group had the least improvement. These results suggest that the bodies of younger people may be better able to convert 5-HTP to serotonin. (Based on my experience, I suspect that the reduced efficiency of 5-HTP conversion in older individuals may be due to a nutritional deficiency or a decrease in the number of serotonin receptor sites in the brain, a normal phenomenon of aging. In Chapter 7 you will learn a little more about other nutrients that support the metabolism of serotonin within the body.)

An essential finding from this year-long study was that L-tryptophan and 5-HTP could be used safely for an extended period of time. The only side effect observed with 5-HTP was mild nausea, which developed in 11 percent of patients in the oldest 5-HTP-treated group.

THE ROLE OF SLEEP IN FIBROMYALGIA

In recent years I have treated scores of patients with fibromyalgia using 5-HTP. My experience has convinced me that most of the positive results can be attributed to 5-HTP's ability to promote a good night's sleep.

My clinical findings are supported by findings in the laboratory. Evidence shows that people with fibromyalgia spend less time in REM sleep and more time in the non-REM sleep stages, especially the shallower, less restorative stages 1 and 2.[8] Due in large measure to these disrupted sleep patterns, people with fibromyalgia wake up feeling tired, worn out, and achy. From my interviews with these patients, I have learned that the better they sleep, the better they feel in the morning. Conversely, when they sleep poorly, they wake up feeling awful.

The link between pain levels and sleep quality was shown quite clearly in a recent study conducted at the University of Connecticut School of Medicine.[9] For thirty days, a group of fifty women with fibromyalgia syndrome kept track of their sleep quality, their pain intensity, and the amount of attention they paid to their pain. Each day, using palmtop computers that were programmed to act as "electronic interviewers," the women would enter comments about their previous night's sleep quality within a half-hour of awakening. Then, at randomly selected times throughout the day and evening, the computer would also prompt them to rate their present level of pain. Analysis of the women's comments clearly showed that poor sleep resulted in significantly more pain. What's more, the researchers found that a night of poor sleep was followed by a significantly more painful day, and that a more painful day was followed by a night of even poorer sleep. For victims of fibromyalgia, this vicious cycle makes life a living hell.

5-HTP breaks this cycle. By correcting the basic underlying problem—low serotonin levels—5-HTP promotes sound, restful sleep. When sleep duration is adequate and the quality is high, the body is better able to heal the damage caused by chronic pain. Furthermore, increased serotonin may have a direct role in mitigating the transmission of pain signals. The more serotonin present, the less vulnerable you are to pain.

NATURAL THERAPY FOR FIBROMYALGIA

If you were to visit a traditional physician—one who had at least heard of fibromyalgia syndrome, anyway—there is a good chance that you would come away with a prescription for one of the various antidepressants. Amitriptyline is often prescribed, not because it lifts mood (although that can be a plus when you suffer from constant, chronic pain) but because it promotes deep sleep. However, it also causes many bothersome side effects, such as weight gain, dry mouth, and disturbed thinking. Other medications prescribed for this condition include antihistamines such as diphenhydramine (Benadryl) and antianxiety drugs such as alprazolam (Xanax). Some evidence exists to support the concept of using a combination of antidepressants such as fluoxetine (Prozac) plus amitriptyline.[10] The Italian investigators I mentioned earlier also noted better results when they combined 5-HTP with an MAO inhibitor.[11]

Remember that studies on the combination of 5-HTP with antidepressants are conducted under strict clinical conditions and under the watchful eye of the researchers. Often, too, these involve patients with severe depression that did not respond to other treatments. I strongly caution my patients not to self-medicate with 5-HTP if they are also taking any other serotonin-active drug, especially an MAO inhibitor or an SSRI.

I believe that 5-HTP is a better alternative to these synthetic drugs or their combinations. 5-HTP works to relieve the syndrome the same way prescription drugs do, by increasing serotonin to promote sleep and tone down sensitivity to pain. But it does so without the risk of serious side effects (and at a much lower cost—a real advantage when you're dealing with a chronic, possibly lifelong condition).

In most cases, I recommend that my patients with fibromyalgia try taking 100 mg of 5-HTP three times a day. This regimen helps to prevent pain throughout the course of the day while promoting healthy sleep patterns at night. Generally, it takes about four weeks for the maximum benefit of 5-HTP to occur. That's because it takes a while for brain cells to adjust the number of serotonin receptors in response to the increased levels of serotonin in the synapses.

5-HTP is certainly effective on its own. However, there are steps you can take to achieve even better results more quickly. Because fibromyalgia causes such a wide range of symptoms, combination therapy is a rational approach. In my clinical experience I have found that the combination of 5-HTP (100 mg), St.-John's-wort extract (300 mg, 0.3 percent hypericin content), and magnesium (200 to 250 mg) three times daily works better than any of these products alone.

Lab studies show that many patients with fibromyalgia (or with chronic fatigue syndrome, a related disorder I'll discuss in a moment) have low magnesium levels.[12] Magnesium supplementation enhances the treatment of both conditions. Its benefits appear to result, at least in part, from its positive impact on serotonin function.[13] I'll have more to say about that in the next chapter.

Use of 5-HTP and selected supplements is part of an overall fibromyalgia treatment plan. Taking steps to improve your sleep patterns is also of value. Try to establish a regular bedtime and stick to it. (Even losing an hour of sleep can exacerbate symptoms, as many people with fibromyalgia discover to their dismay when daylight saving time begins!)

Gentle daily aerobic exercise can help. Apparently the benefits have more to do with the improved quality of sleep that results from exercise, not from any workout your muscles get. Avoid strenuous or high-impact exercise, such as jogging or weight lifting. If possible, try "aquacise," in which you do your workout in the water to avoid putting too much stress on muscles and joints.

Eat a diet low in fats and simple sugars, and avoid any foods that you know are likely to trigger headaches. Cut out caffeine.

Since stress can make symptoms of fibromyalgia worse, do what you can to reduce emotional and physical upset. Pace yourself. Practice relaxation techniques. Resist the temptation to do too much. If an episode of symptoms becomes too much to take, don't try to fight it. Call in sick, go home early, decline the party invitation, and give yourself the rest you deserve.

Power Over Pain:

PHYLLIS'S STORY

Phyllis, a fifty-three-year old woman, thought she was "coming apart at the seams." For nearly fifteen years she had suffered from a nearly constant ache that suffused her every muscle. Some days she could barely drag herself out of bed. When she awoke in the morning she would lie for a minute with her eyes open, registering the signals from her rebellious body. As soon as she moved her arm or shifted her leg—sometimes if she even blinked her eyes—she would sense the presence of pain. "I think I know how a termite-infested house feels," she remarked. "It's as if there's something inside me, gnawing away at my very foundation."

She had made the rounds of doctors. Most of them conducted extensive (and expensive) tests but could find nothing specific to point to and say, "Aha! There's the problem." Others identified her condition as arthritis, an infection, or (in one frightening instance) cancer. Another stopped just shy of accusing her of being a furtive drug abuser. One doctor had said her problem was "all in her head" and referred her to a psychiatrist, who put her on a tricyclic antidepressant. The drug helped only a little. Phyllis began to wonder if maybe she was just imagining things.

One day while waiting to see her gynecologist she was leafing through a health magazine and spotted an article about fibromyalgia syndrome. She almost wept with relief when she recognized her sufferings in the description of its symptoms. "At last, my enemy had a name," Phyllis said.

Meanwhile, though, the problem kept getting worse. She had to give up working full time in her job at a travel agency. Normally a meticulous housekeeper, she had stopped trying to keep the house in order, and she seldom cooked for her family anymore. "It's just too exhausting," she said. "I fill a pot of water to start making my famous linguine and the effort just wipes me out."

Her symptoms were also making things hard on her husband, Bob, and their children. The times when she had to skip visits with relatives or decline invitations to holiday picnics and family outings were too numerous to count. One night her husband said that the worst part of her illness, for him, was that they'd had to give up going to monthly square dances, where they'd first met almost twenty years before.

At that point Phyllis decided she had had enough and that she was going to "lick this thing." Firmly believing that conventional medicine had no answers for her, she undertook a quest that led her to many different alternative medical practitioners—acupuncturists, massage therapists, bodyworkers, and naturopathic physicians. She felt a little better, but she still had frequent migraine headaches. Her muscles were tender and aching, she slept poorly at night, and during the day she constantly battled feelings of irritability and depression.

By the time she came to see me, she was taking no fewer than twenty different nutritional supplements and herbal products. Many of these were useful in promoting general health, and a few addressed some various aspects of fibromyalgia, but her regimen was not really focused on her specific biochemical needs. I explained to Phyllis about the role of serotonin in the body and spelled out for her the problems that can result from low serotonin levels. I recommended taking 50 mg of 5-HTP three times a day for the first two weeks and increasing that to 100 mg three times per day thereafter. In addition, I prescribed St.-John's-wort extract, 300 mg three times daily; a high-potency multiple vitamin and mineral formula; additional vitamin E (400 IU daily) and vitamin C (500 mg three times a day), plus magnesium at a dose of 250 mg three times a day and a daily tablespoon of flaxseed oil.

I saw Phyllis again two months after she started this regimen, and she was a changed woman. Her first words to me were, "I want to tell you that I have never slept as well as I have for the past month." As she put it, her whole body seemed to have shed the "crust" that was making her stiff and tight. She felt lighter, as if an invisible weight had been lifted off her. Her energy level had risen "a thousand percent," and she was about to go back to work full time. And she and Bob had a date to go square-dancing the following Saturday.

"It is unbelievable," she said. "I finally feel like I have found the answer to what has been wrong with me for all of these years."

In For the Long Haul:

VIRGINIA'S STORY

The importance of taking 5-HTP for long periods as a treatment for fibromyalgia is demonstrated in the experience of my patient Virginia, a forty-two-year-old homemaker. Like Phyllis and other victims of fibromyalgia, she had bounced around from doctor to doctor looking for a cure for her chronic pain. She tried ibuprofen, but it severely upset her stomach. Over the past five years she had tried antidepressants, special diets, and supplements. At one point a doctor told her that her condition was "incurable" and that she should just "learn to live with it."

Unwilling to accept that she was a hopeless case, she came to see me. As I reviewed her chart I noticed that she reported having strong cravings for sweets, suffered from frequent headaches, and had trouble falling and staying asleep. Clearly Virginia was experiencing a number of manifestations of the serotonin deficiency syndrome, although fibromyalgia was her main complaint.

I recommended the same "triple therapy" as prescribed for Phyllis and described above.

After years of living without hope, Virginia was clearly excited about the prospect that this approach would relieve her pain. But at her six-week checkup she told me that while her mood was better and her sleep had improved, she hadn't noticed much improvement in her pain at all. I reminded her that sometimes it takes a while for 5-HTP to produce the physiological changes in the serotonin receptors in her body needed to alleviate pain syndromes, including fibromyalgia. I encouraged her to stay the course.

She did. When I saw her again after three months of therapy, Virginia proclaimed herself cured of her "incurable" illness. I urged her to continue with her treatment program for three more months, after which I had her stop the St.-John's-wort extract and the extra magnesium, and shift the 5-HTP dosage to 150 mg at bedtime.

After another three months on this regimen, I suggested she might be able to stop taking 5-HTP. At my recommendation, she gradually tapered off over the course of a month. But a few days after she had stopped 5-HTP completely, she called to report that her fibromyalgia had come back "with a vengeance." I told her to start taking it again immediately (150 mg at bedtime), and she experienced complete relief after only three nights. Currently she is taking a maintenance dose of 50 mg each night and has reported no further symptoms.

Chronic Fatigue Syndrome

Chronic fatigue syndrome (CFS) is a condition very similar to fibromyalgia. In fact, about 70 percent of patients diagnosed with fibromyalgia also meet all of the diagnostic criteria for CFS.[14] Some experts argue that these two syndromes may actually be the same medical condition.

The chief difference between the two in terms of their diagnostic criteria is that fibromyalgia involves musculoskeletal pain (but not necessarily fatigue), while CFS causes overwhelming fatigue (but not necessarily pain). In many cases, the diagnosis you receive depends to a great extent on the type of doctor you consult. Confronted with a patient exhibiting the same pattern of symptoms, a rheumatologist or orthopedic specialist is more likely to call the condition fibromyalgia, while an internist will be more likely to use the term CFS—assuming, of course, that these doctors recognize the syndromes as real in the first place.

Given this relationship between the two syndromes, it will not surprise you to learn that treatment with 5-HTP can be very helpful for people suffering from CFS. It is possible that 5-HTP is even more beneficial in dealing with CFS, because chronic fatigue involves even more severe types of sleep pattern disturbances.

CFS can be a very debilitating disorder. People with this condition can become totally exhausted after even the slightest exertion. As one patient told me, "I can't brush my teeth in the morning without feeling like I've spent my entire energy budget for the day." People with CFS suffer from a range of nonspecific symptoms, including weakness, muscle aches and pains, excessive sleep, insomnia, malaise (a general "blah" feeling), fever, sore throat, tender lymph nodes, impaired memory, trouble concentrating, and depression. As the term *chronic* indicates, CFS can persist for years.

Although CFS was first identified as a legitimate illness a decade ago, we still do not know what causes it. The symptoms of the syndrome resemble those seen in other conditions, including infection with viruses (such as the Epstein-Barr virus). However, there is no single virus that is found in all people who have CFS.

Many experts believe that in some cases a virus, stress, or some other health problem can cause the immune system to go into high gear and to stay revved up even after the danger has passed. As a result of this immune-system overactivity, certain chemicals (known as immune activating factors) may remain in the blood-stream. These factors, in high doses, are known to cause fatigue.

The Centers for Disease Control and Prevention (CDC) esti-mates that CFS affects more than four out of every thousand Americans over the age of eighteen. Other researchers believe the rate is even higher, and that more than five million people in this country currently suffer from CFS. Like fibromyalgia, CFS affects more women than men; about 80 percent of cases occur in women, especially white women twenty-five to forty-five years old. However, CFS can strike men and women of any ethnic origin and at any age.

As with fibromyalgia, there is no specific diagnostic test for CFS. The diagnosis is made according to the pattern of symptoms present (Table 6.3) and after other possible diseases have been ruled out. The patient must experience profound fatigue and other symptoms for at least six months to qualify for a diagnosis of CFS.

**Table 6.3: CDC Diagnostic Criteria for
            Chronic Fatigue Syndrome**

- Major criteria
  - New onset of fatigue causing 50 percent reduction in activ-ity for at least six months
  - Exclusion of other illnesses that can cause fatigue
- Minor criteria
  - Presence of at least eight of eleven symptoms, or
  - Presence of six or more symptoms plus at least two of the three signs

  Symptoms:
  - Mild fever
  - Recurrent sore throat

- Painful lymph nodes
- Muscle weakness
- Muscle pain
- Prolonged fatigue after exercise
- Recurrent headache
- Migratory joint pain
- Neurological or psychological complaints
  - Sensitivity to bright light
  - Forgetfulness
  - Confusion
  - Inability to concentrate
  - Excessive irritability
  - Depression
- Sleep disturbance (hypersomnia or insomnia)
- Sudden onset of symptom complex

Signs:
- Low-grade fever
- Sore throat (nonexudative pharyngitis)
- Palpable or tender lymph nodes

Like fibromyalgia victims, many patients with CFS have made the rounds of doctors and have tried an amazing—and discouraging—range of treatments for their condition. There are no known medications that completely and permanently address the symptoms of CFS. Some drugs can address specific complaints in the short term. For example, antidepressants are often prescribed for CFS patients, although usually at lower doses than those needed to treat depression. Other conventional treatments include pain relievers, such as aspirin and the nonsteroidal anti-inflammatory drugs. Some patients are given potent benzodiazepines to relieve anxiety (such as Xanax, Ativan, and BuSpar) or to promote sleep

(Klonopin, Halcion, or Restoril). Of course, these drugs have the potential to cause serious adverse effects, and the benzodiazepines can cause sleep disturbances, depression, and other complications. Some physicians have prescribed calcium channel blockers, immune suppressants, beta-blockers, allergy medications, even anticancer drugs. However, no clear-cut evidence has been found that any of these do any good for patients with CFS, and their potential to cause long-term adverse reactions is distressingly high.

From my clinical experience, I firmly believe that the best approach to CFS involves restoring the body's natural healing powers. The first goal is to improve the restful and restorative quality of sleep. That's where 5-HTP comes in.

Treatment of chronic fatigue syndrome requires identifying and addressing as many of the factors involved as possible. I tell my patients that both their energy level and their emotional state are determined primarily by two things: their internal focus and their physiology. By "internal focus" I mean the images they hold before their mind's eye and the habitual way they talk to themselves. By "physiology" I refer to bodily factors such as posture, breathing, nutritional state, and hormonal balance. I suggest that people with CFS follow a set of guidelines for maximizing energy levels (see box below).

How to Boost Your Energy

- Think positively.
- Become a student of optimism.
- Eliminate consumption of sugar, caffeine, and alcohol.
- Breathe deeply, from the diaphragm, and hold in the body in an upright posture.
- Drink at least 48 ounces of water daily.

- Practice a gentle but energy-building exercise, such as tai chi or yoga. Try to perform this exercise for at least thirty minutes, five times per week.
- Support proper body chemistry by taking the following supplements:
  - High potency multiple vitamin and mineral supplement (see Chapter 7)
  - Vitamin C: 500 to 1,000 mg three times daily
  - Vitamin E: 200 to 400 IU daily
  - Flaxseed oil: One tablespoon daily
  - Thymus extract: 750 mg of the crude polypeptide fraction once or twice daily
  - Magnesium: 150 to 300 mg three times daily
- Increase serotonin levels by taking the following:
  - 5-HTP: 150 to 300 mg at bedtime
  - St.-John's-wort extract (0.3 percent hypericin content): 300 mg three times per day

Premenstrual Syndrome

PMS is a set of physical and emotional symptoms that develop anywhere from two to fourteen days before menstruation.[15] Typical symptoms include decreased energy, tension, irritability, depression, headache, altered sex drive, breast pain, backache, abdominal bloating, and swelling (edema) in the joints, especially the fingers and ankles.

Although virtually all women of childbearing age have menstrual periods, PMS does not affect everyone. Only about 30 to 40 percent of menstruating women will experience PMS, and it tends to be more common, and the symptoms more severe, among women in their thirties and forties.[16] Apparently the body becomes more vulnerable to symptoms with advancing age. Fortunately, in most cases, symptoms are relatively mild. But for about one out of ten women who experience PMS, the symptoms can be quite severe, leading to depression, irritability, and severe mood swings. When the condition goes beyond a physical complaint to include these signs of mental problems, doctors refer to it as a psychiatric diagnosis known as premenstrual dysphoric disorder.[17] The word *dysphoria* means the opposite of *euphoria*.

Table 6.4: Signs and Symptoms of Premenstrual Syndrome

- Behavioral
  - Nervousness, anxiety, and irritability
  - Mood swings and mild to severe personality change
  - Fatigue, lethargy, and depression
  - Sleep disturbances
- Physical
  - Abdominal bloating
  - Diarrhea and/or constipation
  - Change in appetite (usually craving of sugar) and weight gain
  - Tender and enlarged breasts
  - Uterine cramping
- General
  - Headache
  - Backache
  - Acne
  - Edema of fingers and ankles
  - Altered libido

Scientists are not exactly sure what causes PMS or why some women are more vulnerable to it than others. The syndrome is no doubt related to the intense hormonal changes that the body undergoes during the menstrual cycle. Compared with their non-PMS-experiencing counterparts, women who suffer from PMS tend to have higher estrogen levels and lower plasma progesterone levels five to ten days before the onset of bleeding. This hormonal imbalance may contribute to PMS by causing any or all of the following:

- Reduced manufacture of serotonin
- Reduced ability of the body to make use of vitamin B_6
- Increased secretion of aldosterone, a steroid secreted by the adrenal glands
- Increased secretion of prolactin (a hormone secreted by the pituitary gland that regulates production of milk by the breasts)
- Impaired liver function

PMS is also more common among women who have had children, whose pregnancies were complicated by such problems as toxemia, or who experience pain and cramping with their periods. It is also more likely to develop if you consume caffeine or alcohol, if you do not exercise, and if there is a lot of stress in your life. Diet also plays a key role (see box on page 224).

There clearly is a two-way relationship between PMS and depression. Depression is a common symptom in many cases of PMS, and PMS symptoms are typically more severe in depressed women.[19] The common link between the conditions appears to be a decrease in the brain level of serotonin. Evidence for this association comes from the fact that women with PMS who eat a low-tryptophan diet experience very severe PMS symptoms, particularly irritability.[20] As you recall, the body needs tryptophan to produce 5-HTP, which in turn gets converted to serotonin.

PMS: "Poor Menu" Syndrome?

Women suffering from PMS typically eat a diet that is even worse than the standard American diet. Research shows that, compared to symptom-free women, PMS patients consume:

- 62 percent more refined carbohydrates
- 275 percent more refined sugar
- 79 percent more dairy products
- 78 percent more sodium
- 53 percent less iron
- 77 percent less manganese
- 52 percent less zinc[18]

Many conventional physicians are quick to prescribe antidepressants as a treatment for PMS, especially Prozac and other drugs that affect the serotonin system. In my view, 5-HTP is more likely to provide even greater benefits than these drugs. 5-HTP raises serotonin levels, of course, but it also offers another advantage: It raises levels of the body's natural pain fighters, the endorphins. Research shows that the increased ratio of estrogen to progesterone found in many PMS sufferers can result in lower endorphin levels.[21] Taking 5-HTP can counteract the effects of this imbalance, leading to reduced pain, improved mood, and an overall better ability to get through the day.

If you suffer from PMS—especially if depression is a significant part of your symptoms—I recommend giving 5-HTP a try. Take 50 to 100 mg of 5-HTP three times a day. Also follow the key dietary recommendations below to support proper brain chemistry and hormone levels in women with PMS.

Table 6.5: Dietary Strategies for Reducing PMS Symptoms

Strategy	Purpose
Reduce the intake of meat and other animal foods while increasing the amount of whole grains, beans, and vegetables	Improves the estrogen-to-progesterone ratio, which reduces the severity of PMS symptoms
Reduce the intake of fat	Lower-fat diet helps lower estrogen levels
Eliminate sugar	Low-sugar diet reduces levels of circulating estrogens
Reduce exposure to environmental estrogens (that is, doses of estrogen that enter your body through hormone-dosed poultry and livestock, as well as foods treated with pesticides and herbicides)	Environmental estrogens can bind to estrogen receptors and can increase the estrogen-to-progesterone ratio
Increase the intake of soy foods	Soy contains phytoestrogens—plant compounds with antiestrogenic activity (reduces the effects of excess estrogen)
Eliminate caffeine	Caffeine intake is directly related to the severity of PMS symptoms, especially breast tenderness and the presence of fibrocystic breast disease
Keep salt intake low	Reducing salt helps relieve water retention and bloating associated with PMS

I also recommend taking appropriate levels of vitamin B_6 and magnesium (see guidelines in Chapter 7). Several double-blind studies confirm that these nutrients can significantly reduce symptoms, particularly depression, among women with PMS.[22]

Parkinson's Disease

Parkinson's disease results from damage to the nerves in the area of the brain that is responsible for controlling muscle tension and movement. The damaged cells are the ones needed to produce the neurotransmitter called dopamine. Over time the disease causes gradually worsening muscle tremors, stiffness, and weakness. Eventually it leads to rigid posture, slow movements, and a shuffling walk. Parkinson's strikes fifty thousand people each year. It is more prevalent in older people, affecting about one out of 250 people over age forty and one in 100 people over age sixty.[23] Men are more likely to develop Parkinson's than women.

The disease usually begins as a slight tremor of one hand, arm, or leg. In the early stages the tremors are more apparent while the person is at rest, such as while sitting or standing, and are less noticeable when the hand or limb is being used. A typical early symptom of Parkinson's disease is "pill-rolling," in which the person appears to be rolling a pill back and forth between the fingers.

As the disease progresses, symptoms get worse. The tremors and weakness affect the limbs on both sides of the body. The hands and the head may shake continuously. The person may walk with stiff, shuffling steps. In many cases, the disease causes a permanently rigid, stooped posture and an unblinking, fixed expression. Eventually the loss of muscle control makes it impossible for people with Parkinson's to take care of themselves or handle routine daily tasks, such as feeding and clothing themselves. Over time the person's speech may become slower and more hesitant, and handwriting becomes increasingly cramped, but the person's mental abilities are usually not affected until late in the disease. Not surprisingly, many people with Parkinson's are also clinically depressed.

There is no cure for Parkinson's, but there is effective treatment. Many people respond very well to a drug called Sinemet. This drug contains two key ingredients: levodopa and carbidopa. Levodopa, or L-dopa, is the "middle step" in the conversion of the amino acid tyrosine into dopamine. Carbidopa is a drug that works by ensuring that more L-dopa is converted to dopamine within the brain, where it is needed, and not within the other tissues of the body. The net result is a significant increase in dopamine. If you read the book *Awakenings* by Oliver Sacks (or saw the movie version starring Robin Williams and Robert De Niro), you may remember the vivid portrayal of a man who was virtually immobilized by Parkinson's and who responded miraculously to treatment with L-dopa.

Warning

Treatment for Parkinson's requires use of prescription medications. Levodopa is usually very effective and is usually the first agent prescribed. Other drugs that may be of value in enhancing dopamine include bromocriptine and amantadine. Certain medications can also help control tremors.

While 5-HTP may be helpful as a supplement to standard treatment for Parkinson's, *5-HTP should never be used alone in these patients*. Increasing serotonin without increasing dopamine can cause symptoms, especially rigidity, to get worse.[25] Parkinson's patients should not take 5-HTP until they have first consulted a physician.

Also, many Parkinson's patients are given a drug called Eldepryl (selegiline). This drug is an MAO inhibitor that prevents the breakdown of dopamine. Patients taking Eldepryl should not take 5-HTP at the same time, since there is a significant risk that this combination can raise serotonin to excessively high levels.[26]

But the improvement that results from Sinemet comes with a price in the form of serious side effects, including depression and insomnia. These adverse effects may arise in part because L-dopa increases dopamine while reducing serotonin. For this reason, adding 5-HTP to the regimen can significantly improve mood and enhance the quality of sleep. In addition, 5-HTP may improve the physical symptoms of the disease to a small extent.[24]

About nine out of ten people with Parkinson's disease suffer from profound depression. In my clinical experience, supplementing standard Parkinson's treatment (that is, Sinemet) with 5-HTP can produce tremendous improvements in mood.

Research supports this concept. A study conducted by Dr. Richard Mayeux and colleagues at Columbia University examined the effect of 5-HTP in seven Parkinson's disease patients who were receiving treatment with Sinemet.[27] The initial dose of 5-HTP was 75 mg. Over the next four months the dose was increased by 25 mg every three days (up to a maximum of 500 mg per day) until the patients reported relief of their depression. At different intervals, the patients were asked to assess their symptoms of depression using the Hamilton scale. As Table 6.6 shows, the results were impressive.

Table 6.6: The Effect of 5-HTP on Depression Associated with Parkinson's Disease

Patient #	5-HTP (mg/day)	Hamilton Score (Before 5-HTP)	Hamilton Score (After 5-HTP)
1	125	22	11
2	75	14	3
3	100	21	13
4	100	12	6
5	500	18	22
6	300	18	7
7	100	17	13

Six of the seven patients dramatically responded to 5-HTP; these improvements are reflected by a significant drop in the severity of their depression according to the Hamilton scale ratings. Five of the six people who responded to 5-HTP needed daily doses of only 75 to 125 mg. The one patient who did not get better (who in fact got worse) was taking a high dose, 500 mg of 5-HTP; it would appear that there are some Parkinson's patients who simply may not benefit from this approach. Clearly, however, in most cases, 5-HTP supplementation is a very good idea in patients with Parkinson's disease taking Sinemet.

The Self Reclaimed:

BILL'S STORY

One of the most dramatic improvements I have ever witnessed in my years of clinical practice involved Bill, a fifty-six-year-old man with Parkinson's disease.

By the time Bill visited my office, the disease had caught him pretty tightly in its grip. Although Parkinson's can strike at any time after age forty, it is rare to see the disease so advanced in a man as young as Bill. Because he could not walk without assistance, he was accompanied by his wife, Ellen, and his daughter Jennifer at his elbow. During my interview, I asked Bill about his medical history. His gruff, curt answers made me aware that Bill was severely depressed and frustrated by his physical condition. He had lost virtually all muscle function. For the past two years he had been unable to dress or feed himself, and he needed help just to go to the toilet. He was taking Sinemet, but it didn't seem to be helping much.

Then a strange thing happened: In the middle of our conversation, Bill suddenly nodded off. His wife apologized, saying that Bill had not been sleeping well for months. In hindsight, I was glad he dozed off, because it gave me a chance to talk to his family. That was when I learned about the true impact that Bill's disease was having on these loving, caring—and frightened—women.

They told me that before Parkinson's struck, Bill had been an active and dynamic individual, a man of pride, independence, and strength. He had founded a successful auto parts business and had served several terms in the Washington State legislature. He had been a loving husband and a doting father. He loved the outdoors and took the family on countless hiking and camping trips into the wilds around Mt. Olympus and Mt. Rainier.

But with the onset of the disease, Bill changed in dramatic ways. "It's not just the loss of control over his body, as bad as that is," Ellen said with tears in her eyes. "His whole mood has changed. It's like the disease has eaten away at his personality." Sadly she and Jennifer described how Bill had become emotionally—and even physically—abusive. No matter what they did to help him, no matter how supportive they tried to be, he would lash out at them. The more dependent he became, the angrier and more sarcastic was his tone. They knew deep down that Bill was reacting to his loss of self-reliance, to the tragic loss of his freedom. His very image of himself as a man had crumbled into dust. He felt powerless, weak, and useless. His spirit was dying.

But they were also sad for themselves, because their lives and their relationship with their beloved Bill had also disintegrated. They were hurt and confused, unable to explain why he should treat them so poorly. They had brought Bill to me to seek help for his condition, yes, but they also were hoping to find answers for themselves as well.

I was deeply touched by the agony of their situation. I told them as honestly as I could that I did not know if I would be able to relieve the physical deterioration of Parkinson's disease. But, I said, I could definitely help with his mood. I recommended a diet low in protein but high in complex carbohydrates and suggested supplementation with a high-potency multiple vitamin and mineral formula designed for optimal nutrition. I also prescribed 200 mg of 5-HTP at bedtime. I also suggested he take *Ginkgo biloba* extract, 80 mg three times a day, to enhance the effects of the 5-HTP. I emphasized, too, that Bill had to continue to take his Sinemet exactly as prescribed.

A week after the visit I got a call from Ellen. She was ecstatic. For the first time in months, Bill was able to feed himself again. With obvious relief, Ellen told me how Bill was once again showing signs of his old self. Naturally, I felt a little overwhelmed by this news. I asked if I could speak to Bill, and she laughed. "No, you can't," she said. "He's out taking a walk!" A week later I saw this remarkable transformation for myself. Bill walked into my office—he was not exactly strolling in, but he was moving without holding on to Ellen's arm. He still had the telltale tremors of Parkinson's disease, but the problem was limited to trembling of the hands and to the characteristic "pill-rolling" gesture. In our conversation he showed the gentle, humorous, even courtly manner that his family had missed so terribly in the past months.

In looking back over this experience, I could not identify any single aspect of his treatment that was most responsible for the improvement. Rather, the results came from the right combination of strategies. Using 5-HTP and the other natural approaches no doubt helped lift Bill's mood. By fine-tuning Bill's brain chemistry, some of the physical obstacles were removed so that the active ingredients in Sinemet could do their jobs more effectively. Seeing signs of improvement in himself also contributed to Bill's determination to keep getting better. Success fueled success.

Was this a miracle? I don't think it stretches the definition of the term much to agree that it was.

Seizure Disorders

In the past few years, a significant amount of research on 5-HTP has focused on its potential use in the treatment of various seizure disorders.[28] The most well-known type of seizure disorder is epilepsy, but there are other types as well, many of them quite rare. In general, studies show that 5-HTP is not of value in the treatment of epilepsy, but it can be useful in other types of diseases that cause the involuntary, jerky, irregular muscle spasms known as myoclonus. Even if you don't have a seizure disorder, you may have experienced a benign form of myoclonus—it's that sudden jerk or spasm of the limbs that sometimes happens just before you fall asleep.

The best response to 5-HTP has been seen in people who have *intention myoclonus,* a form of muscle spasm that occurs when the person intends to move the limb. For example, if the person starts to reach for a book on a shelf, the arm might suddenly extend in an unexpected, jerky motion. Intention myoclonus often results from damage to the brain due to lack of oxygen, which might occur following a stroke or heart attack, drug overdose or allergy, severe asthma attack, or exposure to chemicals. (The scientific name for seizures of this type is *postanoxic* ["after lack of oxygen"] *myoclonus.*)

A study by Dr. Melvin Van Woert and colleagues at the Mount Sinai School of Medicine in New York showed that most patients with intention myoclonus experienced dramatic improvement in their symptoms after taking 5-HTP plus carbidopa.[29] (As mentioned earlier, carbidopa is a drug that blocks the enzyme that converts tryptophan into 5-HTP in the blood. This may allow more conversion to take place in the brain and thus may help increase brain serotonin levels. Although research is still going on to determine the role of carbidopa in this process, many experts conclude that it is not necessary to take carbidopa to enjoy the benefits of 5-HTP.[30]) The authors attributed the results to the fact that serotonin depletion seems to be an underlying cause of seizures, and that restoring serotonin supplies can bring them under control. In addition, these investigators noted that 5-HTP plus carbidopa might also help patients with other forms of seizure disorder, such as progressive myoclonus epilepsy, essential myoclonus, palatal myoclonus, and Friedreich's ataxia.

In a 1983 article, Dr. Van Woert noted that treatment of

seizures with this substance could produce results in some cases where nothing else worked. As he stated, "Some helpless bedridden patients dramatically improved to the extent that they could walk again and resume independent living." Because of the phenomenal results Dr. Van Woert was seeing, he contacted nearly 130 pharmaceutical companies, hoping to inspire one of them to develop 5-HTP as a drug for myoclonus. Yet each one turned him down. They acknowledged that the results were impressive but claimed that it wasn't "financially feasible" for them to develop 5-HTP because there were too few people suffering from myoclonus.[31]

Something very good came out of Dr. Van Woert's efforts and those of the National Organization for Rare Disorders: passage of the Orphan Drug Act. This legislation provides financial incentives for drug companies to develop treatments for conditions that affect fewer than two hundred thousand people in the United States. Such small patient populations make it hard for drug companies to recoup their costs after spending the millions of dollars needed to develop a drug for commercial sale.

5-HTP was the first compound to be evaluated as an orphan drug by the Pharmaceutical Manufacturers Association's Commission on Drugs for Rare Diseases. On June 11, 1982, the commission declared that the "orphan drug" 5-HTP was a valuable treatment for postanoxic myoclonus. Despite this declaration, none of the members of the Pharmaceutical Manufacturers Association volunteered to "adopt" 5-HTP.

Fortunately for people with myoclonus, or those suffering from a number of other serious conditions, 5-HTP is now available as an over-the-counter product.

Key Points of This Chapter

- 5-HTP produces excellent results as a treatment for fibromyalgia and chronic fatigue syndrome, due in large measure to its improvement of sleep quality and mood.

- Combining 5-HTP with St.-John's-wort extract and magnesium provides better results than using any of the three alone.
- 5-HTP can relieve symptoms of PMS, especially in women who experience premenstrual depression.
- 5-HTP can help relieve the depression and insomnia associated with Parkinson's disease, but in these patients it must be used in combination with standard Parkinson's treatments (such as Sinemet).
- 5-HTP can help with some types of seizure disorders, sometimes producing dramatic results.
- If you suffer from chronic muscle pain or overall body pain, see your physician for a medical evaluation.
- People with Parkinson's disease should not stop taking or adjust dosages of any prescribed medication, nor should they begin taking 5-HTP, without first consulting their physician.
- People who are taking Eldepryl (selegiline) should not take 5-HTP.

CHAPTER 7

5-HTP AND NUTRITIONAL SUPPLEMENTS AND HERBAL MEDICINES: ENHANCING FACTORS

As you have seen throughout this book, 5-HTP is one of the stars of the intricate chemical ballet going on inside your brain. But like all stars, 5-HTP performs best when it has help from a supporting cast and a behind-the-scenes crew. To convert 5-HTP into serotonin efficiently, and to use serotonin effectively, your body needs a good supply of several other essential nutrients. In addition, a number of herbal medicines can complement and enhance the benefits of 5-HTP (besides providing benefits of their own). This chapter describes these products and explains the steps you can take to get the most out of your 5-HTP treatment.

Nutritional Supplementation and 5-HTP

The brain is a complex chemical factory that requires a constant supply of raw materials. A dietary deficiency of even a single key nutrient can alter brain function. As you have learned throughout this book, serotonin plays a critical role in many important body functions. To maintain healthy levels of this essential neurotransmitter, your diet must contain adequate levels of several B vitamins (Table 7.1) as well as an important mineral, magnesium.

Table 7.1: The B Vitamins Needed for Serotonin Synthesis

- Vitamin B_1 (thiamine)
- Vitamin B_2 (riboflavin)
- Vitamin B_3 (niacin)
- Vitamin B_6 (pyridoxine)
- Vitamin B_{12}
- Biotin
- Pantothenic acid
- Folic acid

B VITAMINS, THIAMINE, AND BRAIN FUNCTION

A recent study on vitamin B_1 (thiamine) involved 120 young female adults who took either 50 mg of thiamine or a placebo each day for two months.[1] The researchers evaluated the women's mood, memory, and reaction times both before and after treatment. The women who took thiamine reported significant improvements in their mood scores, ratings of clearheadedness, and reaction times. In contrast, no improvements were noted for these measurements among the placebo group.

One of the interesting aspects of this study was that, prior to treatment, the subjects were found to have normal levels of thiamine in their blood. In other words, they were not thiamine-deficient. Even so, taking a thiamine supplement provided benefits by boosting their brain activity. Such findings raise questions about whether the currently accepted "normal" values for thiamine are indeed adequate. If not, nutritionists will need to reassess the recommended dietary allowance (RDA) of this important substance.

The first symptoms of a subclinical nutritional deficiency are usually psychological. In other words, if you aren't getting high enough levels of a vitamin or mineral, you will probably first notice the problem not as a physical complaint but as a small change in the way you think or behave. No doubt many Americans, particularly elderly individuals in hospitals or nursing homes, suffer from mental impairment or depression that would improve with better nutrition. Thiamine is one of the nutrients that can help.

FOLIC ACID AND VITAMIN B_{12}

Folic acid and vitamin B_{12} are two nutrients that usually work as a team. Your body needs adequate levels of both to convert 5-HTP into serotonin.

Folic acid deficiency is the single most common nutritional problem in the world, and depression is the most common symptom of inadequate folic acid. Studies show that up to 35 percent of depressed patients are deficient in folic acid.[2] This percentage is probably even higher among the elderly. Studies have found that the rate of folic acid deficiency among elderly patients admitted to a psychiatric ward ranges from 35 percent to nearly 93 percent.[3]

Vitamin B_{12} deficiency is a less common problem, but it too can contribute to depression, especially in the elderly.[4] It is not surprising, then, that correcting deficiencies in folic acid and vitamin B_{12} can result in a dramatic improvement in mood.

If 5-HTP is to be converted to serotonin, it is absolutely critical to have folic acid and vitamin B_{12} available in sufficient quantities.[5] What's more, in order for 5-HTP or conventional antidepressant drugs to have the effects I've noted, a sufficient supply of folic acid and vitamin B_{12} must be present in the body. Without these nutrients, the body can't produce or make use of serotonin and other brain chemicals as efficiently. One of the reasons some people fail to respond to drugs, or to 5-HTP for that matter, may be that their levels of these nutrients are just too low.

In most cases, daily doses of 800 micrograms (mcg) of folic acid and 800 mcg of vitamin B_{12} should be adequate to prevent deficiencies. Always take folic acid supplements along with vitamin B_{12}; doing so prevents folic acid from masking a vitamin B_{12} deficiency.

VITAMIN B_6

Vitamin B_6 is also critically involved in the manufacture and activity of all the monoamine neurotransmitters, including serotonin. What's more, if vitamin B_6 levels are low, then more 5-HTP will get converted in the liver into another substance, kynurenine, which means less will be available to make serotonin. As is the case with its sister substances folic acid and vitamin B_{12}, levels of B_6 are typically quite low in depressed patients and in women taking birth control pills or conjugated estrogens such as Premarin.[6] In my view, many people who suffer from depression may simply have low levels of vitamin B_6. In such cases, supplementation may allow them to avoid having to take prescription antidepressants. I have seen very good results when depressed patients with low B_6 levels supplement their diet with a daily dose of B_6 of 50 mg to 100 mg.

VITAMIN B_3 (NIACIN)

Niacin plays a role in over fifty different chemical reactions in the body. Enzymes that contain niacin are involved in energy production; metabolism of fat, cholesterol, and carbohydrates; and the manufacture of many body compounds, including the sex hormones and adrenal hormones.

Your body can produce its own supply of niacin. The process is much the same as the one that results in 5-HTP: Enzymes in the liver convert molecules of the amino acid tryptophan into niacin. But if you have low serotonin levels, this conversion process is a little like robbing Peter to pay Paul. It's a better idea to boost niacin levels through diet or supplementation so that your liver can use its limited supply of tryptophan to churn out 5-HTP instead.

If you are taking 5-HTP, your daily intake of niacin should be between 50 and 100 mg. Be aware that doses above 100 mg may sometimes produce a "niacin flush," a temporary redness and warmth that results from increased blood flow to the skin.

MAGNESIUM

Magnesium is essential for many of the activities that go on inside the cells of your body, including energy production, protein formation, and reproduction. Magnesium participates in more than three hundred enzymatic reactions, particularly those that produce energy. When your magnesium levels are adequate, your energy level is high.

Unfortunately, though, magnesium deficiency is extremely common among Americans. The RDA for magnesium is 350 mg for men and 280 mg for women. However, the actual average daily intake of magnesium by healthy adults in the United States is only 143 to 266 mg. The main cause of the problem is the choice of foods in the diet. Magnesium occurs abundantly in whole foods. The best dietary sources of magnesium are legumes, tofu, seeds, nuts, whole grains, and green leafy vegetables. Fish, meat, milk, and most fruits are low in magnesium. But most Americans eat processed foods, and, as you probably know, food processing strips away large quantities of vital nutrients, including magnesium.

Magnesium supplementation has been shown to be an effective treatment for a large number of common health conditions (Table 7.2).[7]

Table 7.2: Conditions Shown to Benefit from Magnesium Supplementation

- Acute myocardial infarction
- Angina
- Asthma and chronic obstructive pulmonary disease
- Cardiac arrhythmias
- Cardiomyopathy
- Cardiovascular disease
- Congestive heart failure
- Diabetes
- Eosinophilia-myalgia syndrome
- Fatigue
- Fibromyalgia
- Glaucoma
- Hearing loss
- High blood pressure
- Hypoglycemia
- Intermittent claudication
- Kidney stones
- Low HDL-cholesterol levels
- Migraine
- Mitral valve prolapse
- Osteoporosis
- Pregnancy complications (toxemia, premature delivery, and others)
- Premenstrual syndrome and dysmenorrhea
- Stroke

DOSAGE RECOMMENDATIONS FOR MAGNESIUM

As is the case with tryptophan, trying to consume adequate amounts of magnesium through diet alone can be a challenge. For most people I recommend supplementing the diet with 6 mg of magnesium per kilogram (2.2 pounds) of body weight. Thus a 110-pound person would take 300 mg, a 154-pound person would take 420 mg, and a 200-pound person would take 540 mg.

In general, magnesium is very well tolerated. Be aware, however, that taking magnesium can sometimes cause loose stools. To minimize this problem, divide the daily dose into thirds and take the divided dose with meals.

Warning

People with kidney disease or severe heart disease (such as high-grade atrio-ventricular block) should not take magnesium or potassium unless under direct supervision by a physician. These substances can cause electrolyte disturbances and can alter heart contractions.

Some Practical Advice

In addition to the guidelines I've given for use of B vitamins and magnesium, I offer three primary practical recommendations for nutritional supplementation to ensure that you get the most out of taking 5-HTP. I call these recommendations my "foundation program," because they provide a solid nutritional basis on which to build a healthier way of life.

RECOMMENDATION #1: TAKE A HIGH-QUALITY MULTIPLE
VITAMIN AND MINERAL FORMULA

The recommendations in Table 7.3 provide an optimum intake
range that will guide you in selecting a high-quality supplement.

Table 7.3: Dose Ranges for Vitamins and Minerals

Product	Range for Adults	Comments
VITAMINS		
Biotin	100–300 mcg	
Choline	10–100 mg	
Folic acid	400 mcg	
Inositol	10–100 mg	
Niacin	50–100 mg	
Niacinamide	10–30 mg	
Pantothenic acid	25–100 mg	
Vitamin A (from beta-carotene)	5,000–25,000 IU	
Vitamin A (retinol)	5,000 IU	Women of childbearing age should not take more than 2,500 IU of retinol daily; higher doses may contribute to birth defects.
Vitamin B_1 (thiamine)	10–100 mg	
Vitamin B_{12}	400 mcg	
Vitamin B_2 (riboflavin)	10–50 mg	
Vitamin B_6 (pyridoxine)	25–100 mg	
Vitamin C (ascorbic acid)	100–1,000 mg	It may be easier to take vitamin C separately.
Vitamin D	100–400 IU	Elderly people in

		nursing homes living in northern latitudes should take doses in the higher range.
Vitamin E (d-alpha tocopherol)	100–800 IU	It may be more cost-effective to take vitamin E separately.
Vitamin K (phytonadione)	60–300 mcg	

MINERALS

Boron	1–6 mg	
Calcium	250–1,250 mg	Women at risk of or suffering from osteoporosis may require a separate calcium supplement to achieve higher dosage levels.
Chromium	200–400 mcg	For diabetes and weight loss, dosages of 600 mcg can be used.
Copper	1–2 mg	
Iodine	50–150 mcg	
Iron	15–30 mg	Men and postmenopausal women rarely need supplemental iron.
Magnesium	250–500 mg	
Manganese	10–15 mg	
Molybdenum	10–25 mcg	
Potassium	200–500 mg	
Selenium	100–200 mcg	
Silica	1–25 mg	
Vanadium	50–100 mcg	
Zinc	15–45 mg	

RECOMMENDATION #2: TAKE EXTRA ANTIOXIDANTS

Antioxidants are very important in protecting against the development of heart disease, cancer, and other chronic degenerative diseases. In addition, antioxidants are thought to slow down the aging process. Low intake of antioxidants can result in decreased serotonin.[8] Conversely, keeping your antioxidant intake high can help you maintain your serotonin levels. Antioxidants are available in plant foods, especially raw fruits and vegetables.

Extensive research shows that a combination of antioxidants provides greater protection than does taking a high dose of any single antioxidant. Mixtures of antioxidant nutrients appear to work together harmoniously to produce the phenomenon known as synergy, where the whole is greater than the sum of the parts. In other words, when it comes to the benefits of antioxidants, $1 + 1 = 3$.

The two primary antioxidants in the human body are vitamins C and E. Vitamin C is water-soluble, which means it is found in tissues that contain water. In contrast, vitamin E is lipid-soluble, so it is found in tissues that contain fat, such as cell membranes. As a rule, the daily dose of antioxidants should be: vitamin C (ascorbic acid), 500 to 1,500 mg; vitamin E (d-alpha tocopherol), 400 to 800 IU.

A high-potency multiple vitamin and mineral formula contains other nutrients you need to support the activity of antioxidants, such as selenium, zinc, and beta-carotene. If you are taking such a product, be aware of the levels of antioxidants it contains. If the levels are too low, consider taking additional doses separately to hit the suggested target.

RECOMMENDATION #3: TAKE ONE TABLESPOON OF FLAXSEED OIL DAILY

Your body needs a certain intake of fat to function properly. As a rule, though, Americans consume far too much fat in their diet.

At most, no more than 30 percent of your calories should come from fat.

I recommend flaxseed oil not for its fat content but because it contains ingredients known as essential fatty acids. Like the anti-oxidants, these fatty acids, especially linoleic acid and linolenic acid, help your body maintain its normal physiology. The fatty acids are needed to build nerve cells and cell membranes and to produce hormonelike substances called prostaglandins. These important nutrients also help by preventing, or helping you recover from, over sixty life-threatening illnesses, including heart disease, stroke, cancer, autoimmune diseases such as multiple sclerosis and rheumatoid arthritis, skin diseases, and many others.[9]

Low levels of omega-3 oils have also been linked to depression.[10] That's because these oils are critical for the proper function of the brain cells responsible for the production, release, and activity of serotonin and other mood-regulating neurotransmitters. Without omega-3 oils, brain cells can't build the sturdy membranes they need to function. In addition, the oils play a major role in promoting serotonin activity: binding at receptor sites, signal transmission, reuptake, and breakdown by the monoamine oxidase enzyme. Given the many important roles omega-3 fatty acids play in the serotonin system, dietary shortages can dramatically affect behavior, mood, and mental function.

Ideally, we would consume sufficient levels of fatty acids by eating plant foods. However, experts estimate that approximately 80 percent of the American population consume insufficient quantities of essential fatty acids in the diet. This insufficiency presents a serious health threat.

Taking just a tablespoon a day of organic, unrefined flaxseed oil is a sound strategy for restoring the proper level of essential fatty acids. Flaxseed oil is unique because it contains adequate amounts of both alpha-linolenic acid (an omega-3 fatty acid) and linoleic acid (an omega-6 fatty acid). In fact, flaxseed oil is the world's richest source of omega-3 fatty acids, which have long been known to provide protection against cardiovascular disease, inflammation, allergy, and cancer. A whopping 58 percent of the weight of flaxseed oil comes from omega-3 fatty acids. That's more than twice the level of the omega-3 fatty acid found in fish oils.

Herbal Medicines

There are four natural herbal medicines you can take to further enhance the action of 5-HTP: the extracts of St.-John's-wort, *Ginkgo biloba,* passionflower, and ginger.

A Word About Herbal Remedies

Most mainstream American doctors know very little about the value of herbal medicines. This stands in sharp contrast to medical practice in most of the rest of the world, where many physicians rely on herbal products, used alone or in combination with conventional medicine, to improve the health of their patients.

In Germany, for example, *70 percent* of medical doctors regularly prescribe herbal products. What's more, the government-funded health care system reimburses the patient for the costs. Acceptance of herbal treatments came about as a result of efforts by an expert panel, called Commission E, appointed by the German Federal Health Agency. Over the years the commission has prepared more than four hundred monographs evaluating the clinical uses of herbal preparations. Under the commission's charter, an herbal medicine—indeed, any prescription medicine—can be sold in Germany if the evidence shows a *reasonable certainty* that its claims are true. In contrast, the U.S.

Food and Drug Administration requires *absolute proof* of both safety and efficacy.

In the United States, a few herbal-based products, such as laxatives and cough syrups, are available that make claims about the specific conditions they are designed to treat. But the majority of herbal products are marketed only as "food supplements." Manufacturers are not allowed to make any therapeutic claim about the product, no matter how strong the evidence in support of that claim might be. So far the FDA has refused to set up an independent panel that would study herbal medicines, nor has it agreed to create acceptable guidelines for marketing such products. As a result, most consumers and health care professionals in this country are prevented from knowing about—let alone benefiting from—herbal medicine.

Often mainstream doctors dismiss the value of herbal products by saying there is "no scientific evidence" to support their use. A look at the vast—and growing—body of published medical literature shows otherwise. For example, over twenty-five double-blind controlled trials on St.-John's-wort for depression show that this product can be of significant benefit compared to placebo or to conventional antidepressants. Another forty double-blind studies show that *Ginkgo biloba* extract is effective in the treatment of decreased blood flow to the brain. And these medicines produce results with virtually no risk of side effects. That's something that no standard prescription drug can claim.

ST.-JOHN'S-WORT EXTRACT

The fastest-rising star in herbal medicine today is St.-John's-wort extract. For centuries in Germany, this humble herb has been a popular choice for relief of depression. In 1994 Germans took sixty-six million doses of the product as prescribed by their doctors. When the data are tallied, the use of the herb in recent years is expected to be even higher.[11] In Germany, St.-John's-wort extract is the first choice—not an "alternative"—for treatment of depression, prescribed eight times more often than Prozac.

Many double-blind studies show St.-John's-wort is an effective antidepressant.[12] What's more, it is safer to use because it has fewer and much less severe side effects than the standard medications. In a large German study involving 3,250 patients, undesired side effects were reported in 2.43 percent of patients; only 1.45 percent thought the problems were bad enough to discontinue therapy.[13] The most frequently noted side effects were gastrointestinal irritation (0.55 percent), allergic reactions (0.52 percent), fatigue (0.4 percent), and restlessness (0.26 percent). There are no published reports about serious drug interactions or toxicity.

In contrast, more than 20 percent of people taking Prozac—that's over one out of five—complain of headache or nausea (or both). More than 10 percent experience nervousness, insomnia, drowsiness, or diarrhea. The published list of side effects associated with the drug includes nearly fifty other problems, ranging from anxiety and tremor to loss of appetite, excessive sweating, and upper respiratory infection. In preclinical trials, the dropout rate of patients taking Prozac was 15 percent.

Given these numbers, which "alternative" would you choose?

HOW DOES ST.-JOHN'S-WORT EXTRACT WORK?

The German health commission issued its monograph for St.-John's-wort in 1984. That report identified the active ingredient in the herb as hypericin. Originally it was theorized that this substance works as a monoamine oxidase inhibitor. That is, it was thought that hypericin interfered with the enzyme that breaks down molecules of serotonin and other neurotransmitters. With the publication of the official monograph, German companies could legally promote use of the herb for psychiatric disturbances, depressive states, anxiety, or nervous excitement.

Income from sales of the product allowed the manufacturers to sponsor further research. Results of these later studies show that, in fact, hypericin does not appear to work like an MAO inhibitor.[14] Instead the antidepressant effect arises from hypericin's effects on the immune system and from its ability to inhibit serotonin reuptake, a property it shares with Prozac and the other SSRI antidepressants.[15] Other evidence suggests that St.-John's-wort contains additional compounds, such as flavonoids, that may also provide therapeutic benefits.

In addition to its positive impact on the serotonin system, St.-John's-wort improves sleep quality, particularly in elderly subjects.[16] Like 5-HTP, St.-John's-wort extract enhances both REM and deep sleep stages 3 and 4. These benefits occur even when St.-John's-wort is taken in divided doses throughout the day, rather than in a single dose at bedtime. This feature makes it more convenient if you are taking a product that combines 5-HTP and St.-John's-wort extract.

All classes of antidepressant drugs have been shown to enhance the effects of 5-HTP, and vice versa. In my opinion, St.-John's-wort extract is a superior agent to use in combination therapy with 5-HTP because it causes far fewer side effects than antidepressant drugs.

GETTING THE RIGHT PRODUCT

The cover story of *Newsweek* for May 5, 1997, featured St.-John's-wort and bore the title "Natural Prozac—Does It Work?" My answer is, "Yes indeed—if you buy the right product." Unfortunately, nowhere in this otherwise fine article was the reader told what to look for when buying St.-John's-wort extract. I would wager that nine out of ten people who decided to try this product walked out of the health food store with the wrong stuff.

Herbal products come in many different forms and qualities. I strongly urge patients to use products that offer standardized doses or guaranteed potency. These herbal products are formulated to contain specific and consistent levels of key compounds.

In the case of St.-John's-wort extract, it is absolutely essential that you select a product that is guaranteed to have a 0.3 percent hypericin content. Taking 300 mg of such a product three times per day would provide you with the effective dose of hypericin needed for relief of problems associated with low serotonin syndrome. Avoid the alcohol-based tincture or capsules that simply contain the dried herb, unless the label explicitly states that each dose provides 0.3 percent hypericin.

Note

Some companies market brands of 5-HTP that combine other ingredients, including St.-John's-wort extract or magnesium, into a single capsule or pill. The problem with such products is that often the doses of these added ingredients are inadequate to achieve their purpose. For example, an effective dose of St.-John's-wort extract is 900 mg a day; the extract must contain the active ingredient, hypericin, at a concentration of 0.3 percent. However, some brands of 5-HTP tout that they also include St.-John's-wort extract—but at doses of only 10 to 30 mg. These amounts are much too small to do any good.

As is the case when buying any product, read the labels carefully. Make sure the product contains adequate and effective levels of all components.

Ginkgo biloba Extract

Ginkgo is perhaps the single most important herbal medicine in the world. Over four hundred scientific studies attest to the medical usefulness of *Ginkgo biloba* extract.[17] This product has been shown to be especially effective in treating cerebrovascular insufficiency, a condition in which not enough blood gets to the brain. Ginkgo also may help slow down, halt, and even reverse the early stages of Alzheimer's.[18]

What's more, *Ginkgo biloba* extract is a very effective antidepressant, in part because it counteracts one of the major changes in brain chemistry associated with aging: the gradual reduction in the number of serotonin receptor sites. In a way, the loss of these receptors is like loss of tread on a tire. Without these receptors, serotonin cannot get enough "traction" to bind to the nerve cell and keep its important signals moving forward. As a result, the elderly are more susceptible to problems associated with low-serotonin syndrome, including depression, impaired mental function, insomnia, and sleep disturbances. These problems may arise even if, technically speaking, the level of serotonin in the brain is adequate.

Besides increasing the number of serotonin receptors, *Ginkgo biloba* extract may also enhance the effects of 5-HTP by inhibiting the MAO enzyme.[19] A preliminary study found that in patients who took 160 mg of *Ginkgo biloba* extract, MAO inhibition was 30 percent higher after one hour and 50 percent higher after three hours. Normally, patients who take standard MAO inhibitor medications are warned not to use any other antidepressants at the same time, because the combined effects can cause serious complications, including death. But the same problem does not occur with ginkgo, apparently because the herbal product acts in a different (or "atypical") way compared to synthetic MAO inhibitors. Because ginkgo does not interact with other antidepressants, patients can safely enhance their standard antidepressant therapy by taking ginkgo in doses of 80 mg three times daily.[20]

Passionflower

The combination of 5-HTP and passionflower is my preferred treatment for very difficult cases of insomnia, especially in elderly patients. The passionflower (*Passiflora incarnata*), a beautiful and unusual-looking flower, is one of my favorite plants. Native to North, Central, and South America, passionflower was widely used by the Aztecs as a sedative and a pain reliever. Its modern name, however, has a biblical origin, because the structure of the blossom is seen as a reflection of the Crucifixion (the Passion) of Christ. The coronal threads that surround the flower symbolize the crown of thorns; the five stamens are the wounds Christ received; and the three stigmatas represent the nails on the cross.

Although the exact pharmacology of passionflower still remains a mystery, animal studies have confirmed what the Aztecs knew: that it produces a sedative and pain-relieving effect. Like St.-John's-wort and *Ginkgo biloba*, passionflower has been approved by the German health care agency for medicinal use. Its primary indication is for nervous restlessness.

Passionflower's chemical constituents include flavonoids and harma alkaloids such as harmine, harmaline, and passicol.[21] Harmine, originally called telepathine, produces a contemplative state and mild euphoria. In highly concentrated doses, it was used by the Germans in World War II as "truth serum."[22]

Furthermore, several harma alkaloids have been shown to inhibit monoamine oxidase, at least to a mild extent.[23] This action may make passionflower particularly useful when taken in combination with 5-HTP.

My experience with a patient, Alice, convinced me of the value of this approach. Alice, seventy-three years young, achieved striking results after just three nights of taking a bedtime dose of 5-HTP (300 mg), niacin (30 mg), and passionflower extract (300 mg of the extract standardized to contain 2.6 percent flavonoids). What makes her case so interesting was the fact that she had been taking 27 mg (nine 3 mg tablets) of melatonin at bedtime with little, if any, effect. Two weeks of 5-HTP plus niacin also proved a disappointment. But when she added the passionflower, her sleep pattern improved enormously. She dropped off to sleep within minutes after turning in, and she stayed asleep throughout the night. After about a month, Alice reduced the dosage of all these medicines by two thirds and continues to enjoy healthy, restful sleep.

When taking 5-HTP in combination with passionflower for sleep, I recommend starting with 100 mg at bedtime and increasing that to 200 mg after a few days if necessary. You can also take passionflower in one of several forms thirty to forty-five minutes before retiring. Here are the dosage recommendations:

Dried herb (or as tea): 4–8 g

Tincture (1:5): 6–8 ml (1.5–2 tsp)

Fluid extract (1:1): 2–4 ml (0.5–1 tsp)

Dry powdered extract (2.6 percent flavonoids): 300–450 mg

Ginger

Like generations of grandmothers before her, my grandmother knew that ginger was good for an upset stomach. Whenever I came down with a tummyache, she would fix me up with real ginger ale, made from ginger extract. It helped enormously. For thousands of years ginger has been used to soothe nausea, relieve stomachache, and prevent vomiting. Recent scientific studies have confirmed ginger's effectiveness in alleviating gastrointestinal distress. Several double-blind studies show that ginger is effective in treating motion sickness, severe nausea and vomiting in pregnancy, and postoperative nausea and vomiting.[24] In these studies, ginger's effects proved to be as good as or better than typical antinausea medications.

If you are one of the few people who experience mild nausea while taking 5-HTP, you might consider taking ginger at the same time. Nausea is more likely to occur with higher doses of 5-HTP, such as those used for promoting weight loss. Besides treating nausea, ginger can actually speed up the rate at which your body generates heat and burns off calories in the form of fat.[25]

To help control nausea produced by 5-HTP, take 1 to 2 grams of dry powdered ginger in capsule form. Some people get good results simply by drinking ginger tea. To take advantage of the calorie-burning quality of ginger, take 100 mg of a standardized extract that contains 20 percent gingerol three times a day, twenty minutes before meals.

Key Points of This Chapter

- To enhance the effects of 5-HTP and support serotonin synthesis:
  - Take a high-potency multiple vitamin and mineral supplement.
  - Take extra antioxidants.
  - Take one tablespoon of flaxseed oil daily.
- To enhance the effects of 5-HTP for depression:
  - If you are under fifty, take St.-John's-wort extract (0.3 percent hypericin content), 300 mg three times daily.
  - If you are over fifty years of age, take *Ginkgo biloba* extract (24 percent ginkgo flavonglycosides) or ginkgo phytosome, 80 mg three times daily.
- To enhance the effects of 5-HTP for insomnia:
  - Take passionflower according to the dosage recommendation given above.
- If you take niacin supplements, do not take more than 100 mg per day.
- Do not stop taking or adjust dosages of any prescribed medication without first consulting your physician.

CHAPTER 8

ANSWERS TO COMMON QUESTIONS ABOUT 5-HTP

WHAT IS 5-HTP?

5-HTP (short for 5-hydroxytryptophan) is a naturally occurring substance, a form of amino acid, that your body uses to produce important brain chemicals. Your body converts the amino acid tryptophan into 5-HTP, then changes 5-HTP into a neurotransmitter called serotonin. Some of the serotonin is then changed into another important brain chemical, melatonin. Taking supplemental doses of 5-HTP raises your supply of serotonin in a safe, quick, and natural way.

WHAT DOES 5-HTP DO?

By itself, 5-HTP does not produce therapeutic effects. Instead, it serves as the building block (or precursor) for serotonin. Serotonin is a chemical messenger that performs many vital functions. It helps regulate mood, sleep, appetite, energy level, and sensitivity to pain. Maintaining appropriately high levels of serotonin can alleviate depression, improve sleep quality, promote weight loss, increase energy levels, and relieve several kinds of headaches and muscle pains. 5-HTP also raises levels of endorphins, the body's natural defense against stress and mild pain.

HOW CAN I INCREASE MY SEROTONIN LEVEL?

It helps somewhat to eat a diet that contains plenty of foods rich in tryptophan, such as milk, cottage cheese, poultry, eggs, red meats, soybeans, tofu, and nuts, especially almonds. However, it is very difficult to consume enough of these foods to supply all the tryptophan you may need on a daily basis. Also, some of these foods may pose other health hazards that greatly offset any value they have as sources of tryptophan. Many dairy products contain high levels of fat and cholesterol, and red meats increase the risk of cancer and other serious health problems.

Until a few years ago it was possible to take a supplement containing a form of tryptophan called L-tryptophan. This product is no longer widely available due to concerns about possible contamination.

Certain prescription drugs, including Prozac and related antidepressants, increase serotonin activity. But these drugs do not actually increase serotonin levels, and they can cause a wide range of serious side effects.

At this time, the easiest and safest way to increase serotonin is by taking products containing 5-HTP.

WHAT ARE THE POSSIBLE SIDE EFFECTS OF 5-HTP?

Certain cells in the digestive system are sensitive to serotonin. Taking 5-HTP can affect these cells and lead to mild, temporary nausea. The problem is more likely to occur at higher doses, such as those used in treating obesity. For most therapeutic purposes, the standard doses (50 to 100 mg taken three times a day) are not likely to trigger nausea. Even if nausea develops, the feeling usually disappears after a while, usually within a few days to two weeks. To minimize the risk, use enteric-coated 5-HTP capsules. These dissolve in the small intestine, not in the stomach. Also consider taking ginger, a natural antinausea substance.

SHOULD 5-HTP BE TAKEN WITH MEALS OR ON AN EMPTY STOMACH?

That depends on your therapeutic goal. If you are taking 5-HTP to regulate appetite and improve weight control, take the dose on an empty stomach twenty minutes before meals. This will enhance the speed with which 5-HTP enters the brain and undergoes conversion to serotonin. For other purposes, the timing probably doesn't matter very much. Taking small doses three times a day effectively treats various conditions with minimal risk of side effects.

DURING THE DAY I DO NOT EAT MUCH, BUT AT NIGHT I TEND TO EAT CONSTANTLY, FROM DINNERTIME UNTIL I GO TO BED. SHOULD I TAKE 5-HTP THROUGHOUT THE DAY OR JUST AT NIGHT?

My recommendation is to eat nutritious balanced meals throughout the day and use 5-HTP (100 mg) twenty minutes before breakfast, lunch, and dinner. For your evening meal, always eat a fresh salad and load up on low-calorie vegetables. If you still find that you are bingeing at night, then take another 100 mg of 5-HTP immediately after dinner.

AT WHAT AGE IS IT APPROPRIATE TO USE 5-HTP?

When used as directed, 5-HTP can be safe at any age. Some studies show that children receiving 5-HTP as treatment for headaches improve greatly, but you should always consult a physician before giving 5-HTP to a child. 5-HTP may also be a good choice for elderly people.

IS 5-HTP ADDICTIVE?

No. There is no evidence or basis to suggest that people become addicted to using 5-HTP.

DOES 5-HTP AFFECT URINE TESTS?

Doctors sometimes measure levels of a substance called 5-HIAA in the urine. This substance results when serotonin is broken down (metabolized) by the body. Levels of 5-HIAA provide a clue about how much serotonin is present: the higher the 5-HIAA level, the more serotonin.

More and more professions and companies are requiring employees to undergo tests to detect illicit drug use. Because 5-HTP is a naturally occurring substance that works by increasing naturally occurring serotonin, it does not interfere with drug tests, nor does it produce "false positive" readings (results that indicate drug use when no such use has occurred).

SINCE 5-HTP INCREASES MELATONIN, WHICH PROMOTES SLEEPINESS, WHY DOESN'T 5-HTP MAKE ME SLEEPY WHEN TAKEN DURING THE DAY?

5-HTP generally raises the level of all monoamine neurotransmitters, including dopamine and norepinephrine. These chemicals stimulate brain activity and offset the effects of melatonin. More important, the body releases its supply of melatonin only at night. This is true even when increased serotonin results in higher melatonin levels. The melatonin is stored inside a brain gland, waiting for signals from the body's inner clock. As a result, daytime sleepiness due to 5-HTP use is very rare.

CAN MY SEROTONIN LEVELS GET TOO HIGH?

Yes. A condition known as the serotonin syndrome can result if the body produces excessively high levels of serotonin or if the body cannot break down serotonin at a fast enough rate. Symptoms of the serotonin syndrome include confusion, fever, shivering, sweating, diarrhea, and muscle spasms. This syndrome does not occur when 5-HTP and L-tryptophan are taken alone. However, the medical literature contains reports of some cases that developed when L-tryptophan was combined with prescription drugs that inhibit activity by the enzyme (monoamine oxidase, or MAO) that breaks down molecules of serotonin. You should stop taking an MAO inhibitor for at least four weeks before beginning therapy with 5-HTP or any other serotonin-active substance. Also, you should not take 5-HTP at the same time as any other prescription antidepressant, including Prozac, unless supervised by a physician. *If you are taking an MAO inhibitor or another antidepressant, consult with your doctor before using 5-HTP.*

NOW THAT REDUX AND FENFLURAMINE (PART OF FEN-PHEN) HAVE BEEN WITHDRAWN FROM THE MARKET, ARE THERE ANY ALTERNATIVES FOR WEIGHT LOSS?

5-HTP helps curb appetite, especially for carbohydrates, by triggering feelings of fullness (satiety). 5-HTP is a safe natural alternative to prescription weight-loss medications.

SINCE 5-HTP REDUCES SUGAR CRAVINGS, CAN IT ALSO HELP WITH URGES TO ABUSE DRUGS OR ALCOHOL?

Based on the many beneficial effects seen in people taking 5-HTP, scientists hoped that 5-HTP would help promote abstinence from alcohol and drugs. Unfortunately, several double-blind studies have not found that such is the case. However, people with substance abuse problems may benefit from using

5-HTP to relieve underlying depression, which may in turn help them in their other efforts to cope with their addiction problem.

DOES CAFFEINE INTERFERE WITH THE EFFECTS OF 5-HTP?

Yes. Caffeine has been shown to counteract the effects of serotonin. What's more, caffeine leads to lower levels of both serotonin and melatonin, which can disturb sleep and lead to troublesome mood swings. For optimal results with 5-HTP, keep caffeine to a minimum. Better yet, avoid it entirely.

CAN 5-HTP BE USED DURING PREGNANCY?

No studies to date have indicated that 5-HTP is harmful during pregnancy. Still, if a woman who is taking 5-HTP becomes pregnant, the sensible thing to do is stop taking it immediately. If you are taking any medication, consult with your doctor as soon as you learn you are pregnant and find out which products you should stop and which you should continue using.

WHERE CAN I GET 5-HTP?

5-HTP is now available as a nutritional supplement in many health food stores and some pharmacies. It is also available by mail order and through your local compounding pharmacist.

APPENDIX: SOURCES OF 5-HTP

Note: This list is provided for the convenience of readers as a general guide. The list is not complete. Inclusion here is not to be construed as an endorsement of the company or its products.

Country Life
28300-B Industrial Boulevard
Hayward, CA 94545
(800) 851-2200
Fax: (800) 221-6799

Life Enhancement
P.O. Box 751390
Petaluma, CA 94975
(800) 543-3873
Fax: (707) 769-8016
Outside the United States:
(707) 762-6144
Fax: (707) 769-8016
http://www.life-enhancement.com

E-mail: info@life-enhancement.com

LifeLink
750 Farroll Road
Grover Beach, CA 93433
(888) 433-5266
Fax: (805) 473-2803
http://www.lifelinknet.com/
E-mail: lifelink@west.net

Natrol
21411 Prarie St.
Chatsworth, CA 91311
(800) 326-1520

Fax: (818) 739-6001
http://www.natrol.com

Natural Balance
3130 N. Commerce Ct.
Castle Rock, CO 80104-8002
(800) 624-4260
Fax: (303) 688-1591
www.pepworld.com

Nutricology, Inc
400 Preda Street
San Leandro, CA 94577
(800) 545-9960
Fax: (510) 635-6730

Pure Encapsulations, Inc.
490 Boston Post Road
Sudbury, MA 01776
(800) 753-2277
Fax: (888) 783-2277

Solaray, Inc.
P.O, Box 681869
Park City, UT 84068
(801) 655-6000
Fax: (801) 647-3802

Solgar
500 Willow Tree Road
Leonia, NJ 07605
(800) 645-2246
Fax: (888) 645-2246
www.solgar.com

Thorne Research
25820 Highway 2 West
Dover, ID 83825
(800) 228-1966
Fax: (208) 265-2488
http://www.thorne.com

Tri Medica
8321 E. Evans Road Suite 102
Scottsdale, AZ 85260
(602) 998-1041
Fax: (602) 998-1530

Vitamin Research Products, Inc.
3579 Hwy. 50 East, Carson City,
NV 89701
(800) 877-2447
(702) 884-1300
Fax: (800) 877-3292
Fax: (702) 884-1331
http://www.vrp.com
E-mail: mail@vrp.com

The Vitamin Shoppe
4700 Westside Avenue
North Bergen, NJ 07047
(800) 223-1216
Fax: (800) 852-7153

NOTES

Chapter 1

1. K. Turlejski, "Evolutionary ancient roles of serotonin: Long-lasting regulation of activity and development," *Acta Neurobiologiae Experimentalis* 56 (1996): 619–36.

2. National Eosinophilia-Myalgia Syndrome Network, *Frequently Asked Questions* (June 1997), http://www.nemsn.org/ems/html/faq.html.

3. E. M. Kilbourne, "Eosinophilia-myalgia syndrome: Coming to grips with a new illness," *Epidemiologic Review* 14 (1992): 16–36; E. M. Kilbourne et al., "Tryptophan produced by Showa Denko and epidemic eosinophilia-myalgia syndrome," *Journal of Rheumatology* 46 suppl. (1996): 81–88.

4. G. A. Filippini, C. V. L. Costa, and A. Bertazzo, eds., "Recent advances in tryptophan research: Tryptophan and serotonin pathways," *Experimental Biology and Medicine* 398 (1996): 1–762; "Proceedings: Eosinophilia-Myalgia Syndrome: Review and Reappraisal of Clinical, Epidemiologic and Animal Studies Symposium. Washington, D.C., December 7–8, 1994," *Journal of Rheumatology* 46 suppl. (1996): 1–110.

5. E. A. Belongia et al., "An investigation of the cause of the eosinophilia-myalgia syndrome associated with tryptophan use," *New England Journal of Medicine* 323 (1990): 357–65.

6. H. Steinhart et al., "Synthesis and analysis of contaminants in EMS-related tryptophan," *Experimental Biology and Medicine* 398 (1996): 667–75.

7. M. Nicolodi and F. Sicuteri, "Eosinophilia-myalgia syndrome: The role of contaminants, the role of serotonergic setup," *Experimental Biology and Medicine* 398 (1996): 351–57.

8. R. Brown, "Tryptophan metabolism in humans," in O. Hayaishi, Y. Ishimura, and R. Kido, eds., *Biochemical and Medical Aspects of Tryptophan Metabolism* (Amsterdam: Elsevier/North Holland Press, 1980), 227–36.

9. I. E. Magnussen and F. Nielsen-Kudsk, "Bioavailability and related pharmacokinetics in man of orally administered L-5-hydroxytryptophan in a steady state," *Acta Pharmacologica et Toxicologica* 46 (1980): 257–62; I. Magnussen et al., "Plasma accumulation and metabolism of orally administered single-dose L-5-hydroxytryptophan in man," *Acta Pharmacologica et Toxicologica* 49 (1981): 184–89.

10. M. Aviram, U. Cogan, and S. Mokady, "Excessive dietary tryptophan enhances plasma lipid peroxidation in rats," *Atherosclerosis* 88 (1991): 29–43.

11. M. G. Simic, M. al-Sheikhly, and S. V. Jovanovic, "Inhibition of free radical processes by antioxidants tryptophan and 5-hydroxytryptophan," *Bibliotheca Nutritio et Dieta* 43 (1989): 288–89.

12. H. M. van Praag and C. Lemus, "Monoamine precursors in the treatment of psychiatric disorders," in R. J. Wurtman and J. J. Wurtman, eds., *Nutrition and the Brain,* vol. 7 (New York: Raven, 1986), 89–139.

Chapter 2

1. American Psychiatric Association, *Diagnostic and Statistical Manual of Mental Disorders,* 4th ed. (Washington, D.C.: American Psychiatric Association, 1994), 317–93.

2. G. D. Tollefson et al., "Evaluation of suicidality during pharmacologic treatment of mood and nonmood disorders," *Annals of Clinical Psychiatry* 5 (1993): 209–24; A. C. Power and P. J. Cowen, "Fluoxetine and suicidal behaviour," *British Journal of Psychiatry* 161 (1992): 735–41; W. C. Wirshing et al., "Fluoxetine, akathisia, and suicidality: Is there a causal connection?" *Archives of General Psychiatry* 49 (1992) 580–81; W. Creaney, I. Murray, and D. Healy, "Antidepressant-induced suicidal ideation," *Human Psychopharmacology* 6 (1991): 329–32; P. Masand, S. Gupta, and M. Dewan, "Suicidal ideation related to fluoxetine [letter]," *New England Journal of Medicine* 324 (1991): 420; A. J. Rothschild and C. A. Locke, "Re-exposure to fluoxetine after serious suicide attempts by three patients: The role of akathisia," *Journal of Clinical Psychiatry* 52 (1991): 491–93.

3. C. M. Beasley et al., "Fluoxetine and suicide: A meta-analysis of controlled trials of treatment for depression," *British Medical Journal* 303 (1991): 685–92; M. V. Rudorfer, H. K. Manji, and W. Z. Potter, "Comparative tolerability profiles of newer versus older antidepressants," *Drug Safety* 10 (1994): 18–46; R. A. King, R. H. Segman, and G. M. Anderson, "Serotonin and suicidality: The impact of acute fluoxetine administration," *Israel Journal of Psychiatry and Related Sciences* 31 (1994): 271–79.

4. N. Miyakoshi, Y. Nishijima, and H. Shindo, "Distribution and metabolism of L-5-hydroxytryptophan-^{14}C in cat brain after intravenous administration," *Japanese Journal of Pharmacology* 24 (1974): 1424.

5. A. Wirz-Justice, "Theoretical and therapeutic potential of indoleamine precursors," *Japanese Journal of Clinical Medicine* 34 (1976): 3294–302.

6. I. Sano, "L-5-hydroxytryptophan therapy," *Folia Psychiatrica et Neurologica Japonica* 26 (1972): 7–17.

7. S. Takahashi, H. Kondo, and N. Kato, "Effect of L-5-hydroxytryptophan on brain monoamine metabolism and evaluation of its clinical effect in depressed patients," *Journal of Psychiatric Research* 12 (1975): 177–87; J. Fujiwara and S. Otsuki, "Subtype of affective psychosis classified by response on amine precursors and monoamine metabolism," *Folia Psychiatrica et Neurologica Japonica* 28 (1974): 94–100.

8. T. Nakajima, Y. Kudo, and Z. Kaneko, "Clinical evaluation of 5-hydroxy-L-tryptophan as an antidepressant drug," *Folia Psychiatrica et Neurologica Japonica* 32 (1978): 223–30.

9. H. M. van Praag et al., "A pilot study of the predictive value of the probenecid test in application of 5-hydroxytryptophan as antidepressant," *Psychopharmacologia* 25 (1972): 14–21.

10. Van Praag, "A pilot study" (see note 9); H. M. van Praag and J. Korf, "5-hydroxytryptophan as an antidepressant. The predictive value of the probenecid test," *Journal of Nervous and Mental Disease* 158 (1974): 331–37.

11. Van Praag and Korf, "5-hydroxytryptophan" (see note 10); H. M. van Praag and J. Korf, "Serotonin metabolism in depression: Clinical application of the probenecid test," *International Pharmacopsychiatry* 9 (1974): 35–51.

12. W. Pöldinger, B. Calanchini, and W. Schwartz, "A functional-dimensional approach to depression: Serotonin deficiency as a target syndrome in a comparison of 5-HTP and fluvoxamine," *Psychopathology* 24 (1991): 53–81.

13. H. M. van Praag, "Studies on the mechanism of action with serotonin precursors in depression," *Psychopharmacology Bulletin* 20 (1984): 599–602.

14. J. Angst, B. Woggon, and J. Schoepf, "The treatment of depression with L-5-hydroxytryptophan versus imipramine: Results of two open and one double-blind study," *Archiv für Psychiatrie und Nervenkrankheiten* 224 (1977): 175–86.

15. H. M. van Praag, "Management of depression with serotonin precursors," *Biological Psychiatry* 16 (1981): 291–310.

16. T. R. Robie and A. Flora, "Anti-depressant chemotherapy, 1965. Rapid response to serotonin precursor potentiated by Ritalin," *Psychosomatics* 6 (1965): 351–54; M. Nardini et al., "Treatment of depression with

L-5-hydroxytryptophan combined with chlorimipramine, a double-blind study," *International Journal of Clinical Pharmacological Research* 3 (1983): 239–50; J. J. Rousseau, "Effects of a levo-5-hydroxytryptophan-dihydroergocristine combination on depression and neuropsychic performance: A double-blind placebo-controlled clinical trial in elderly patients," *Clinical Therapeutics* 9 (1987): 267–72; J. Mendlewicz and M. B. Youdim, "Antidepressant potentiation of 5-hydroxytryptophan by L-deprenil in affective illness," *Journal of Affective Disorders* 2 (1980): 137–46.

17. J. J. Alino, J. L. Gutierrez, and M. L. Iglesias, "5-hydroxytryptophan (5-HTP) and an MAOI (nialamide) in the treatment of depressions. A double-blind controlled study," *International Pharmacopsychiatry* 11 (1976): 8–15.

18. T. G. Martin, "Serotonin syndrome," *Annals of Emergency Medicine* 28, no. 5 (1996): 520–26.

19. W. F. Byerley et al., "5-hydroxytryptophan: A review of its antidepressant efficacy and adverse effects," *Journal of Clinical Psychopharmacology* 7 (1987): 127–37.

20. Pöldinger, Calanchini, and Schwartz, "A functional-dimensional approach" (see note 12).

21. H. M. van Praag, "Central monoamine metabolism in depressions. I. Serotonin and related compounds," *Comprehensive Psychiatry* 21 (1980): 30–43.

22. J. J. van Hiele, "L-5-hydroxytryptophan in depression: The first substitution therapy in psychiatry?" *Neuropsychobiology* 6 (1980): 230–40.

23. A. C. Pande and M. E. Sayler, "Adverse events and treatment discontinuations in fluoxetine clinical trials," *International Clinical Psychopharmacology* 8 (1993): 267–69.

24. R. Balon et al., "Sexual dysfunction during antidepressant treatment," *Journal of Clinical Psychiatry* 54 (1993): 209–12; M. Herman and D. S. Goldbloom, "Fluoxetine-induced sexual dysfunction," *Journal of Clinical Psychiatry* 42 (1990): 25–27.

25. W. M. Patterson, "Fluoxetine-induced sexual dysfunction," *Journal of Clinical Psychiatry* 54 (1993): 71.

26. L. J. Brandes et al., "Stimulation of malignant growth in rodents by antidepressant drugs at clinically relevant doses," *Cancer Research* 52 (1992): 3796–800.

27. O. Benkert, "Effect of parachlorophenylalanine and 5-hydroxytryptophan on human sexual behavior," *Monographs in Neural Sciences* 3 (1976): 88–93; O. Benkert, "Studies on pituitary hormones and releasing hormones in depression and sexual impotence," *Progress in Brain Research* 42 (1975): 25–36.

28. R. P. Hullin and T. Jerram, "Sexual disinhibition with L-tryptophan," *British Medical Journal* 2 (1976): 1010; G. P. Egan and G. E. Hammad, "Sexual inhibition with L-tryptophan," *British Medical Journal* 2 (1976): 701.

29. H. M. van Praag and C. Lemus, "Monoamine precursors in the treatment of

psychiatric disorders," in R. J. Wurtman and J. J. Wurtman, eds., *Nutrition and the Brain,* vol. 7 (New York: Raven, 1986), 89–139.

30. Van Praag and C. Lemus, "Monoamine precursors" (see note 29); H. M. van Praag et al., "In search of the mode of action of antidepressants: 5-HTP/tyrosine mixtures in depression," *Advances in Biological Psychiatry* 10 (1983): 148–59.

31. Van Praag and C. Lemus, "Monoamine precursors" (see note 29); A. J. Gelenberg and C. J. Gibson, "Tyrosine for the treatment of depression," *Nutrition and Health* 3 (1984): 163–73; C. Gibson and A. Gelenberg, "Tyrosine for depression," *Advances in Biological Psychiatry* 10 (1983): 148–59; H. Beckman, "Phenylalanine in affective disorders," *Advances in Biological Psychiatry* 10 (1983): 137–47.

32. K. Zmilacher, R. Battegay, and M. Gastpar, "L-5-hydroxytryptophan alone and in combination with a peripheral decarboxylase inhibitor in the treatment of depression," *Neuropsychobiology* 20 (1988): 28–35.

33. C. J. Robins and A. M. Hayes, "An appraisal of cognitive therapy," *Journal of Consulting and Clinical Psychology* 61 (1993): 205–14; M. Evans et al., "Differential relapse following cognitive therapy and pharmacotherapy for depression," *Archives of General Psychiatry* 49 (1992): 802–8.

34. R. B. Jarrett and A. J. Rush, "Short-term psychotherapy of depressive disorders: Current status and future directions," *Psychiatry* 57 (1994): 115–32.

35. C. Peterson, M. Seligman, and G. Valliant, "Pessimistic explanatory style as a risk factor for physical illness: A thirty-five-year longitudinal study," *Journal of Personality and Social Psychology* 55 (1988): 23–27; C. Peterson, "Explanatory style as a risk factor for illness," *Cognitive Therapy and Research* 12 (1988): 117–30.

36. S. Weyerer and B. Kupfer, "Physical exercise and psychological health," *Sports Medicine* 17 (1994): 108–16; E. W. Martinsen, "The role of aerobic exercise in the treatment of depression," *Stress Medicine* 3 (1987): 93–100. R. C. Casper, "Exercise and mood," *World Review of Nutrition and Dietetics* 71 (1993): 115–43; D. Carr et al., "Physical conditioning facilitates the exercise-induced secretion of beta-endorphin and beta-lipoprotein in women," *New England Journal of Medicine* 305 (1981): 560–65.

37. D. Lobstein, B. J. Mosbacher, and A. H. Ismail, "Depression as a powerful discriminator between physically active and sedentary middle-aged men," *Journal of Psychosomatic Research* 27 (1983): 69–76.

38. A. Winokur, "Insulin resistance after glucose tolerance testing in patients with major depression," *American Journal of Psychiatry* 145 (1988): 325–30; J. H. Wright et al., "Glucose metabolism in unipolar depression," *British Journal of Psychiatry* 132 (1978): 386–93.

39. M. Werbach, *Nutritional Influences on Mental Illness: A Sourcebook of Clinical Research* (Tarzana, Ca.: Third Line Press, 1991).

Chapter 3

1. R. J. Wurtman and J. J. Wurtman, "Brain serotonin, carbohydrate-craving, obesity, and depression," *Advances in Experimental Medicine and Biology* 398 (1996): 35–41; J. Wurtman and S. Suffes, *The Serotonin Solution* (New York: Fawcett Columbine, 1997).

2. Wurtman and Suffes, *The Serotonin Solution* (see note 1); G. M. Goodwin et al., "Plasma concentrations of tryptophan and dieting," *British Medical Journal* 300 (1990): 1499–1500; I. M. Anderson et al., "Dieting reduces plasma tryptophan and alters brain 5-HTP function in women," *Psychological Medicine* 20, no. 4 (1990): 785–91; B. E. Wolfe, E. D. Metzger, and C. Stollar, "The effects of dieting on plasma tryptophan concentration and food intake in healthy women," *Physiology and Behavior* 61, no. 4 (1997): 537–41.

3. J. E. Blundel and M. B. Leshem, "The effect of 5-HTP on food intake and on the anorexic action of amphetamine and fenfluramine," *Journal of Pharmacy and Pharmacology* 27 (1975): 31–37.

4. T. E. Weltzin, M. H. Fernstrom, and W. H. Kaye, "Serotonin and bulimia nervosa," *Nutrition Reviews* 52 (1994): 399–408.

5. T. E. Weltzin et al., "Acute tryptophan depletion and increased food intake and irritability in bulimia nervosa," *American Journal of Psychiatry* 152 (1995): 1668–71.

6. Weltzin et al., "Acute tryptophan depletion" (see note 5).

7. D. S. Goldbloom, P. E. Garfinkel, R. Katz, and G. M. Brown, "The hormonal response to intravenous 5-hydroxytryptophan in bulimia nervosa," *Journal of Psychosomatic Research* 40, no. 3 (1996): 289–97.

8. F. Ceci et al., "The effects of oral 5-hydroxytryptophan administration on feeding behavior in obese adult female subjects," *Journal of Neural Transmission* 76 (1989): 109–17.

9. C. Cangiano et al., "Effects of 5-hydroxytryptophan on eating behavior and adherence to dietary prescriptions in obese adult subjects," *Advances in Experimental Medicine and Biology* 294 (1991): 591–93.

10. C. Cangiano et al., "Eating behavior and adherence to dietary prescriptions in obese adult subjects treated with 5-hydroxytryptophan," *American Journal of Clinical Nutrition* 56 (1992): 863–67.

11. H. Muller-Fassbender et al., "Glucosamine sulfate compared to ibuprofen in osteoarthritis of the knee," *Osteoarthritis and Cartilage* 2 (1994): 61–69; L. C. Rovati et al., "A large, randomized, placebo-controlled, double-blind study of glucosamine sulfate vs. piroxicam and vs. their association, on the kinetics of the symptomatic effect in knee osteoarthritis," *Osteoarthritis and Cartilage* 2 (suppl. 1) (1994): 56; A. L. Vaz, "Double-blind clinical evaluation of the relative efficacy of ibuprofen and glucosamine sulfate in the management of osteoarthrosis of the knee in outpatients," *Current Medical Research and Opinion* 8 (1982): 145–49.

12. B. Guy-Grand et al., "International trial of long-term dexfenfluramine in obesity," *Lancet* 2 (1989): 1142–44.

13. M. L. Drent et al., "The effect of dexfenfluramine on eating habits in a Dutch ambulatory android overweight population with an overconsumption of snacks," *International Journal of Obesity* 19 (1996): 749–51.

14. R. Davis and D. Faulds, "Dexfenfluramine: An updated review of its therapeutic use in the management of obesity," *Drugs* 52 (1996): 696–724.

15. H. M. Connolly, J. L. Crary, M. D. McGood et al., "Valvular heart disease association with fenfluramine-phentermine," *New England Journal of Medicine* 337, no. 9 (1997): 581–88.

16. L. B. Cannistra, S. M. Davis, and A. G. Bauman, "Valvular heart disease associated with dexfenfluramine [letter]," *New England Journal of Medicine* 337, no. 9 (1997): 636.

17. M. D. Lemonick, "The mood molecule," *Time* 150, no. 13 (1997): 75–82.

18. K. A. Sporer, "The serotonin syndrome. Implicated drugs, pathophysiology and management," *Drug Safety* 13, no. 2 (1995): 94–104.

19. S. Robbins, *Pathologic Basis of Disease* (Philadelphia: W. B. Saunders, 1984), 579–80.

20. G. A. Spiller, *Dietary Fiber in Health and Nutrition* (Boca Raton: CRC Press, 1994).

Chapter 4

1. P. Sheras-Koch and A. Lemley, *The Dream Sourcebook* (Los Angeles: Lowell House, 1996).

2. R. J. Wyatt et al., "Effects of 5-hydroxytryptophan on the sleep of normal human subjects," *Electroencephalography and Clinical Neurophysiology* 30 (1971): 505–9.

3. V. P. Zarcone Jr. and E. Hoddes, "Effects of 5-hydroxytryptophan on fragmentation of REM sleep in alcoholics," *American Journal of Psychiatry* 132, no. 1 (1975): 74–76.

4. A. Irving and W. Jones, "Methods for testing impairment of driving due to drugs," *European Journal of Clinical Pharmacology* 43 (1992): 61–66.

5. H. Denison et al., "Influence of increased adrenergic activity and magnesium depletion on cardiac rhythm in alcohol withdrawal," *British Heart Journal* 72, no. 6 (1994): 554–60.

6. H. P. Landolt et al., "Late-afternoon ethanol intake affects nocturnal sleep and the sleep EEG in middle-aged men," *Journal of Clinical Psychopharmacol-

ogy 16, no. 6 (1996): 428–36; P. M. Thompson et al., "Polygraphic sleep measures differentiate alcoholics and stimulant abusers during short-term abstinence," *Biological Psychiatry* 38, no. 12 (1995): 831–36; H. J. Aubin et al., "Alcohol, sleep and biological rhythms" [in French], *Neurophysiologie Clinique* 23, no. 1 (1993): 61–70.

7. G. Hajak et al., "The influence of intravenous L-tryptophan on plasma melatonin and sleep in men," *Pharmacopsychiatry* 24 (1991): 17–20.

8. C. L. Spinweber et al., "L-tryptophan: Effects on daytime sleep latency and the waking EEG," *Electroencephalography and Clinical Neurophysiology* 55, no. 6 (1983): 652–61; L. A. Steinberg et al., "Tryptophan intake influences infants' sleep latency," *Journal of Nutrition* 122, no. 9 (1992): 1781–91; E. Hartmann, "Effects of L-tryptophan on sleepiness and on sleep," *Journal of Psychiatric Research* 17, no 2 (1982–83): 107–13.

9. C. L. Spinweber, "L-tryptophan administered to chronic sleep-onset insomniacs: Late-appearing reduction of sleep latency," *Psychopharmacology* 90 (1986): 151–55; D. Helmert-Schneider, "Interval therapy with L-tryptophan in severe chronic insomniacs: A predictive laboratory study," *International Pharmacopsychiatry* 16 (1981): 162–73; K. Demisch et al., "Treatment of severe chronic insomnia with L-tryptophan: Results of a double-blind cross-over study," *Pharmacopsychiatry* 20 (1987): 242–44; J. G. Lindsley, E. L. Hartmann, and W. Mitchell, "Selectivity in response to L-tryptophan among insomniac subjects: A preliminary report," *Sleep* 6 (1983): 2467–56; L. J. Fitten, J. Profita, and T. G. Bidder, "L-tryptophan as a hypnotic in special cases," *Journal of the American Geriatrics Society* 33 (1985): 294–97; E. Hartmann, "L-tryptophan: A possible natural hypnotic substance" [editorial], *Journal of the American Medical Association* 230 (1974): 1690–81; E. Hartmann, "L-tryptophan: A rational hypnotic with clinical potential," *American Journal of Psychiatry* 134 (1977): 366–70.

10. F. Ferrero and J. Zahnd, "Tryptophan in the treatment of insomnia in hospitalized psychiatric patients," *Encephale* 3 (1987): 35–37; E. Hartmann, J. G. Lindsley, and C. Spinweber, "Chronic insomnia: Effects of tryptophan, flurazepam, secobarbital, and placebo," *Psychopharmacology* (Berlin) 80 (1983): 138–42; C. C. Brown, N. J. Horrom, and A. M. Wagman, "Effects of L-tryptophan on sleep onset insomniacs," *Waking and Sleeping* 3 (1979): 101–8.

11. R. J. Wyatt, "The serotonin-catecholamine-dream bicycle: A clinical study," *Biological Psychiatry* 5 (1972): 33–64; R. J. Wyatt et al., "Effects of L-tryptophan (a natural sedative) on human sleep," *Lancet* 2 (1970): 842–46.

12. Wyatt, "The serotonin-catecholamine-dream bicycle" (see note 11); C. Guilleminault, H. P. Cathala, and P. Castaigne, "Effects of 5-HTP on sleep of a patient with brain stem lesion," *Electroencephalography and Clinical Neurophysiology* 34 (1973): 177–84; Wyatt et al., "Effects of 5-hydroxytryptophan" (see note 2); A. Autret et al., "Human sleep and 5-HTP. Effects of repeated high doses and of association with benserazide," *Electroencephalography and Clinical Neurophysiology* 41 (1976): 408–13; Zarcone and Hoddes, "Effects of 5-hydroxytryptophan" (see note 3); A. Soulairac and H. Lambinet, "Effect of 5-hydroxytryptophan, a serotonin precursor, on sleep disorders," *Annales Medico-Psychologiques* 1 (1977): 792–98; A. Soulairac and H. Lambinet, "Clinical studies of the effect of the serotonin precursor, L-5-hydroxytryptophan, on sleep disorders," *Schweizerische Rundschau für Medizin Praxis* 77 (1988): 19–23.

13. I. V. Zhdanova et al., "Sleep-inducing effects of low doses of melatonin ingested in the evening," *Clinical Pharmacology and Therapeutics* 57 (1995): 552–58; J. G. MacFarlane et al., "The effects of exogenous melatonin on the total sleep time and daytime alertness of chronic insomniacs: A preliminary study," *Biological Psychiatry* 30 (1991): 371–76; S. P. James et al., "Melatonin administration in insomnia," *Neuropsychopharmacology* 3 (1990): 19–23.

14. R. Nave, R. Peled, and P. Lavie, "Melatonin improves evening napping," *European Journal of Pharmacology* 275 (1995): 213–16.

15. I. Haimov et al., "Sleep disorders and melatonin rhythms in elderly people," *British Medical Journal* 309 (1994): 167; I. Haimov et al., "Melatonin replacement therapy of elderly insomniacs," *Sleep* 18 (1995): 598–603.

16. R. C. Zimmermann et al., "Effects of acute tryptophan depletion on nocturnal melatonin secretion in humans," *Journal of Clinical Endocrinology and Metabolism* 76, no. 5 (1993): 1160–64.

17. D. W. Hudgel, E. A. Gordon, and H. Y. Meltzer, "Abnormal serotonergic stimulation of cortisol production in obstructive sleep apnea," *American Journal of Respiratory and Critical Care Medicine* 152, no. 1 (1995): 186–92; H. S. Schmidt, "L-tryptophan in the treatment of impaired respiration in sleep," *Bulletin Européen de Physiopathologic Respiratoire* 19 (1983): 625–29.

18. D. A. Hanzel, N. G. Proia, and D. W. Hudgel, "Response òf obstructive sleep apnea to fluoxetine and protriptyline," *Chest* 100, no. 2 (1991): 416–21.

19. Schmidt, "L-tryptophan" (see note 17).

20. Hudgel, Gordon, and Meltzer, "Abnormal serotonergic stimulation" (see note 17).

21. D. W. Hudgel and E. A. Gordon, "Serotonin-induced cortisol release in CPAP-treated obstructive sleep apnea patients," *Chest* 111, no. 3 (1997): 632–38.

22. A. Autret et al., "Clinical and polygraphic effects of D,L-5-HTP on narcolepsy-cataplexy," *Biomedicine* 27 (1977): 200–3.

23. J. M. Bouchard and M. Pujol, "5-HTP in clinical sleep disorders in humans," *Psychiatry* 53 (1977): 215; G. De Giorgis et al., "Headache in association with sleep disorders in children: A psychodiagnostic evaluation and controlled clinical study—L-5-HTP versus placebo," *Drugs Under Experimental and Clinical Research* 13 (1987): 425–33.

24. S. T. O'Keeffe, K. Gavin, and J. N. Lavan, "Iron status and restless legs syndrome in the elderly," *Age and Aging* 23 (1994): 200–3.

Chapter 5

1. M. Leone et al., "Beta-endorphin level in lymphocytes of primary headache patients," *Cephalalgia* 5, suppl. 3 (1991): 188–189; P. A. Battistella et al., "Beta-endorphin in plasma and monocytes in juvenile headache," *Headache* 36 (1996): 91–94.

2. N. T. Mathew, "Chronic refractory headache," *Neurology* 43, suppl. 3 (1993): S26–S33; N. T. Mathew, "Transformed migraine," *Cephalalgia* 13, suppl. 12 (1993): 78–83; N. T. Mathew, R. Kurman, and F. Perez, "Drug-induced refractory headache: Clinical features and management," *Headache* 30 (1990): 634–38.

3. G. De Benedittis and R. Massei, "Serotonin precursors in chronic primary headache: A double-blind cross-over study with L-5-hydroxytryptophan vs. placebo," *Journal of Neurosurgical Science* 29 (1985): 239–48.

4. A. Kagaya et al., "Serotonin-induced desensitization of serotonin$_2$ receptors in human platelets via mechanism involving protein kinase C," *Journal of Pharmacology and Experimental Therapeutics* 255 (1990): 305–11.

5. R. W. Kimball, A. P. Friedman, and E. Vallejo, "Effect of serotonin in migraine patients," *Neurology* 10 (1960): 107–11.

6. M. D. Ferrari et al., "Serotonin metabolism in migraine," *Neurology* 33 (1989): 1239–42.

7. L. Fioroni et al., "Platelet serotonin pathway in menstrual migraine," *Cephalalgia* 16 (1966): 427–30; J. W. Lance et al., "5-hydroxytryptamine and its putative aetiological involvement in migraine," *Cephalalgia* 9 suppl. (1989): 7–13.

8. F. Titus et al., "5-hydroxytryptophan versus methysergide in the prophylaxis of migraine: Randomized clinical trial," *European Neurology* 25 (1986): 327–29.

9. Battistella et al., "Beta-endorphin" (see note 1); A. R. Genazzani et al., "Central regulation of circulating beta-endorphin: Possible implication in headache treatments," *Cephalalgia* 5, suppl. 3 (1985): 102–3; A. R. Genazzani et al., "Effects of 5-HTP with and without carbidopa on plasma beta-endorphin and pain perception," *Cephalalgia* 6 (1986): 642–45.

10. Titus et al., "5-hydroxytryptophan versus methysergide" (see note 8).

11. F. Sicuteri, "5-hydroxytryptophan in the prophylaxis of migraine," *Pharmacological Research Communications* 5 (1972): 213–18; F. Sicuteri, "The ingestion of serotonin precursors (L-5-hydroxytryptophan and L-tryptophan) improves migraine," *Headache* 13 (1973): 19–22.

12. Battistella et al., "Beta-endorphin" (see note 1); G. De Giorgis et al., "Headache in association with sleep disorders in children: A psychodiagnostic evaluation and controlled clinical study—L-5-HTP versus placebo," *Drugs Under Experimental and Clinical Research* 13 (1987): 425–33; M. Santucci et al., "L-5-hydroxytryptophan versus placebo in childhood migraine prophylaxis: A double-blind crossover study," *Cephalalgia* 6 (1986): 155–57; G. Longo et al., "Treatment of essential headache in developmental age with L-5-HTP (crossover double-blind study versus placebo)," *Pediatria Medica e Chirurgica* 6 (1984): 241–45.

13. De Giorgis, "Headache in association" (see note 12).

14. Battistella et al., "Beta-endorphin" (see note 1); I. Fettes et al., "Endorphin levels in headache syndromes," *Headache* 25 (1984): 37–39; M. Leone et al., "Beta-endorphin level in lymphocytes of primary headache patients," *Cephalalgia* 11, suppl. 11 (1991): 188–89.

15. De Giorgis, "Headache in association" (see note 12).

Chapter 6

1. S. Cooke, "Is it fibromyalgia: Making progress with this difficult-to-diagnose disease," *Caring Magazine* 13, no. 1 (1997), http://www.hsc.missouri.educ/fibro/isitfms.html.

2. F. Sicuteri, "The ingestion of serotonin precursors (L-5-hydroxytryptophan and L-tryptophan) improves migraine," *Headache* 13 (1973): 19–22.

3. M. Nicolodi and F. Sicuteri, "Fibromyalgia and migraine, two faces of the same mechanism. Serotonin as the common clue for pathogenesis and therapy," *Advances in Experimental Medicine and Biology* 398 (1996): 373–79.

4. M. Nicolodi and F. Sicuteri, "Eosinophilia-myalgia syndrome: The role of contaminants, the role of serotonergic setup," *Experimental Biology and Medicine* 398 (1996): 351–57.

5. I. Caruso et al., "Double-blind study of 5-hydroxytryptophan versus placebo in the treatment of primary fibromyalgia syndrome," *Journal of International Medical Research* 18 (1990): 201–9.

6. P. S. Puttini and I. Caruso, "Primary fibromyalgia syndrome and 5-hydroxy-L-tryptophan: A 90-day open study," *Journal of International Medical Research* 20 (1992): 182–89.

7. Nicolodi and Sicuteri, "Eosinophilia-myalgia syndrome" (see note 4).

8. K. P. White and M. Harth, "An analytical review of 24 controlled clinical trials for fibromyalgia syndrome (FMS)," *Pain* 64 (1996): 63–68.

9. G. Afflect et al., "Sequential daily relations of sleep, pain intensity, and attention to pain among women with fibromyalgia," *Pain* 68 (1996): 363–68.

10. D. Goldenberg et al., "A randomized, double-blind crossover trial of fluoxetine and amitriptyline in the treatment of fibromyalgia," *Arthritis and Rheumatism* 39 (1996): 1852–59.

11. Nicolodi and Sicuteri, "Fibromyalgia and migraine" (see note 3).

12. T. J. Romano and J. W. Stiller, "Magnesium deficiency in fibromyalgia syndrome," *Journal of Nutritional Medicine* 4 (1994): 165–67; I. M. Cox, M. J. Campbell, and D. Dowson, "Red blood cell magnesium and chronic fatigue syndrome," *Lancet* 337 (1991): 757–60.

13. G. Abraham, "Management of fibromyalgia: Rationale for the use of magnesium and malic acid," *Journal of Nutritional Medicine* 3 (1992): 49–59; J. T. Hicks, "Treatment of fatigue in general practice: A double-blind study," *Clinical Medicine* 1 (1964): 85–90.

14. D. Buchwald and D. Garrity, "Comparison of patients with chronic fatigue syndrome, fibromyalgia, and multiple chemical sensitivities," *Archives of Internal Medicine* 154 (1994): 2049–53.

15. K. T. Barnhart, E. W. Freeman, and S. J. Sondheimer, "A clinician's guide to the premenstrual syndrome," *Medical Clinics of North America* 79 (1995): 1457–72.

16. American Psychiatric Association, *Diagnostic and Statistical Manual of Mental Disorders*, 4th ed. (Washington, D.C.: American Psychiatric Association, 1994), 716.

17. M. Steiner, "Premenstrual dysphoric disorder: An update," *General Hospital Psychiatry* 18 (1996): 244–50.

18. G. E. Abraham, "Nutritional factors in the etiology of the premenstrual tension syndromes," *Journal of Reproductive Medicine* 28 (1983): 446–64.

19. Barnhart, Freeman, and Sondheimer, "A clinician's guide" (see note 15).

20. D. B. Menkes, D. C. Coates, and J. P. Fawcett, "Acute tryptophan depletion aggravates premenstrual syndrome," *Journal of Affective Disorders* 32, no. 1 (1994): 37–44; S. Steinberg et al., "Tryptophan in the treatment of late luteal phase dysphoric disorder: A pilot study," *Journal of Psychiatry and Neuroscience* 19, no. 2 (1994): 114–19; R. Sayegh et al., "The effect of a carbohydrate-rich beverage on mood, appetite, and cognitive function in women with premenstrual syndrome," *Obstetrics and Gynecology* 84, no. 4, part 1 (1995): 520–28.

21. F. Facchinetti et al., "Oestradiol/progesterone imbalance and the premenstrual syndrome," *Lancet* 2 (1983): 1302.

22. Abraham, "Nutritional factors" (see note 18); M. K. Berman et al., "Vitamin B$_6$ in premenstrual syndrome," *Journal of the American Dietetics Association* 90 (1990): 859–61; J. Kliejnen, G. Ter Riet, and P. Knipschild, "Vitamin B$_6$ in the treatment of premenstrual syndrome: A review," *British Journal of Obstetrics and Gynaecology* 97 (1990): 847–52; F. Facchinetti et al., "Oral magnesium successfully relieves premenstrual mood changes," *Obstetrics and Gynecology* 78 (1991): 177–81.

23. R. Berkow et al., *The Merck Manual of Medical Information, Home Edition* (Whitehouse Station, N.J.: Merck Research Laboratories, 1997), 315.

24. R. Mayeux et al., "The relationship of serotonin to depression in Parkinson's disease," *Movement Disorders* 3 (1988): 237–44; J. Bastard, J. L. Truelle, and J. Emile, "Effectiveness of 5-hydroxytryptophan in Parkinson's disease," *Nouvelle Presse Medicale* 5 (1976): 1836–37; V. I. Sano and K. Taniguchi, "L-5-hydroxytryptophan (L-5-HTP) therapy in Parkinson's disease," *Morbidity and Mortality Weekly Report* 114 (1972): 1717–19.

25. T. N. Chase, L. K. Ng, and A. M. Watanabe, "Parkinson's disease: Modification by 5-hydroxytryptophan," *Neurology* 22 (1972): 479–84.

26. J. Mendlewicz and M. B. Youdim, "Antidepressant potentiation of 5-hydroxytryptophan by L-deprenil in affective illness," *Journal of Affective Disorders* 2 (1980): 137–46.

27. Mayeux et al., "The relationship of serotonin to depression" (see note 24).

28. M. R. Pranzatelli et al., "A controlled trial of 5-hydroxy-L-tryptophan for ataxia in progressive myoclonus epilepsy," *Clinical Neurology and Neurosurgery* 98 (1996): 161–64; P. Trouillas et al., "Levorotatory form of 5-hydroxytryptophan in Friedreich's ataxia: Results of a double-blind drug-placebo cooperative study," *Archives of Neurology* 52 (1995): 456–60; K. Wessel et al., "Double-blind crossover study with levorotatory form of hydroxytryptophan in patients with degenerative cerebellar diseases," *Archives of Neurology* 52 (1995): 451–55; M. R. Pranzatelli et al., "Neuropharmacology of progressive myoclonus epilepsy: Response to 5-hydroxy-L-tryptophan," *Epilepsia* 36 (1995): 783–91; P. Trouillas, F. Brudon, and P. Adeleine, "Improvement of cerebellar ataxia with levorotatory form of 5-hydroxytryptophan," *Archives of Neurology* 45 (1988): 1217–22.

29. M. H. Van Woert et al., "Serotonin and myoclonus," *Monographs in Neural Sciences* 3 (1976): 71–80.

30. Wessel et al., "Double-blind crossover study" (see note 28).

31. M. H. Van Woert, "Myoclonus and L-5-hydroxytryptophan (L-5-HTP)," *Progress in Clinical and Biological Research* 127 (1983): 43–52.

Chapter 7

1. D. Benton, R. Griffiths, and J. Haller, "Thiamine supplementation, mood and cognitive functioning," *Psychopharmacology* (Berlin) 129 (1997): 66–71.

2. R. Crellin, T. Bottiglieri, and E. H. Reynolds, "Folates and psychiatric disorders: Clinical potential," *Drugs* 45 (1993): 623–36; M. W. P. Carney et al., "Red cell folate concentrations in psychiatric patients," *Journal of Affective Disorders* 19 (1990): 207–13; E. Reynolds et al., "Folate deficiency in depressive illness," *British Journal of Psychiatry* 117 (1970): 287–92.

3. W. E. Thornton and B. P. Thornton, "Geriatric mental function and folic acid: A review and survey," *Southern Medicine Journal* 70 (1977): 919–22; F. Abalan et al., "Frequency of deficiencies of vitamin B_{12} and folic acid in patients admitted to a geriatric-psychiatry unit," *Encephale* 10 (1984): 9–12.

4. S. L. Kivela, K. Pahkala, and A. Eronen, "Depression in the aged: Relation to folate and vitamins C and B_{12}," *Biological Psychiatry* 26 (1989): 209–13.

5. M. Botez et al., "Effect of folic acid and vitamin B_{12} deficiencies on 5-hydroxyindoleacetic acid in human cerebrospinal fluid," *Annals of Neurology* 12 (1982): 479–84.

6. C. Russ et al., "Vitamin B_6 status of depressed and obsessive-compulsive patients," *Nutritional Reports International* 27 (1983): 867–73; M. Carney, D. Williams, and B. Sheffield, "Thiamin and pyridoxine lack in newly admitted psychiatric patients," *British Journal of Psychiatry* 135 (1979): 249–54; J. W. Stewart et al., "Low B_6 levels in depressed outpatients," *Biological Psychiatry* 19 (1984): 613–16.

7. M. T. Murray, *Encyclopedia of Nutritional Supplements* (Rocklin, Ca.: Prima, 1996).

8. A. Castano et al., "Changes in the turnover of monoamines in prefrontal cortex of rats fed on vitamin E-deficient diet," *Journal of Neurochemistry* 58 (1992): 1889–95.

9. Murray, *Encyclopedia* (see note 7).

10. J. R. Hibbeln and N. Salem, "Dietary polyunsaturated fatty acids and depression: When cholesterol does not satisfy," *American Journal of Clinical Nutrition* 62 (1995): 1–9.

11. P. A. G. De Smet and W. Nolen, "St. John's wort as an antidepressant," *British Medical Journal* 313 (1996): 241–42.

12. E. Ernst, "St. John's wort, an antidepressant? A systematic, criteria-based review," *Phytomedicine* 2 (1995): 67–71.

13. H. Woelk, G. Burkard, and J. Grunwald, "Benefits and risks of the hypericum extract LI 160: Drug monitoring study with 3,250 patients," *Journal of Geriatric Psychiatry and Neurology* 7, suppl. 1 (1994): S34–S38.

14. H. M. Thiede and A. Walper, "Inhibition of MAO and COMT by hypericum extracts and hypericin," *Journal of Geriatric Psychiatry and Neurology* 7, suppl. 1 (1994): S54–S56.

15. B. Thiele, I. Brink, and M. Ploch, "Modulation of cytokin expression by hypericum extract," *Journal of Geriatric Psychiatry and Neurology* 7, suppl. 1 (1994): S60–S62; S. Perovic and W. E. G. Muller, "Pharmacological profile of hypericum extract: Effect of serotonin uptake by postsynaptic receptors," *Arzneimittel-Forschung* 45 (1995): 1145–48.

16. H. Schulz and M. Jobert, "Effects of hypericum extract on the sleep EEG in older volunteers," *Journal of Geriatric Psychiatry and Neurology* 7, suppl. 1 (1994): S39–S43.

17. J. Kleijnen and P. Knipschild, "Ginkgo biloba," *Lancet* 340 (1992): 1136–39; J. Kleijnen and P. Knipschild, "Ginkgo biloba for cerebral insufficiency," *British*

Journal of Clinical Pharmacology 34 (1992): 352–58; B. Schneider, "Ginkgo biloba extract in peripheral arterial diseases: Meta-analysis of controlled clinical studies," *Arzneimittel-Forschung* 42 (1992): 428–36.

18. F. V. DeFeudis, ed., *Ginkgo Biloba Extract (Egb 761): Pharmacological Activities and Clinical Applications* (Paris: Elsevier, 1991); B. Hofferberth, "The efficacy of Egb761 in patients with senile dementia of the Alzheimer type: A double-blind, placebo-controlled study on different levels of investigation," *Human Psychopharmacology* 9 (1994): 215–22.

19. H. L. White, P. W. Scates, and B. R. Cooper, "Extracts of ginkgo biloba leaves inhibit monoamine oxidase," *Life Sciences* 58 (1996): 1315–21.

20. DeFeudis, *Ginkgo Biloba Extract* (see note 18); H. Schubert and P. Halama, "Depressive episode primarily unresponsive to therapy in elderly patients: Efficacy of Ginkgo biloba (Egb 761) in combination with antidepressants," *Geriatrische Forschung* 3 (1993): 45–53.

21. J. Bruneton, *Pharmacognosy, Phytochemistry, Medicinal Plants* (Paris: Lavoisier, 1995).

22. W. Embodden, *Narcotic Plants* (New York: Collier, 1980).

23. E. Speroni and A. Minghetti, "Neuropharmacological activity of extracts from Passiflora incarnata," *Planta Medica* 57 (1988): 488–91.

24. D. Mowrey and D. Clayson, "Motion sickness, ginger, and psychophysics," *Lancet* 1 (1982): 655–57; J. J. Stewart et al., "Effects of ginger on motion sickness susceptibility and gastric function," *Pharmacology* 42 (1991): 111–20; W. Fischer-Rasmussen et al., "Ginger treatment of hyperemesis gravidarum," *European Journal of Obstetrics, Gynecology and Reproductive Biology* 38 (1990): 19–24; M. E. Bone et al., "Ginger root—a new antiemetic. The effect of ginger root on postoperative nausea and vomiting after major gynecological surgery," *Anaesthesia* 45 (1990): 669–71.

25. Y. Kano, Q. N. Zong, and K. Komatsu, "Pharmacological properties of galenical preparation. XIV. Body temperature retaining effect of the Chinese traditional medicine 'goshuyu-to' and component crude drugs," *Chemical and Pharmaceutical Bulletin* 39 (1991): 690–92; T. P. D. Eldershaw et al., "Pungent principles of ginger (Zingiber officinale) are thermogenic in the perfused rat hind limb," *International Journal of Obesity* 16 (1992): 755–63; C. J. K. Henry and S. M. Piggott, "Effect of ginger on metabolic rate," *Human Nutrition, Clinical Nutrition* 41C (1985): 89–92.

INDEX

ABOUT THE AUTHOR

Michael Murray, N.D., is one of the world's leading authorities on natural medicine. He serves on the faculty and board of trustees of Bastyr University in Seattle, Washington, and is a consultant to the health food and natural health industries. He is the author of many books, including *The Healing Power of Herbs*, *The Healing Power of Foods*, *Natural Alternatives to Over-the-Counter and Prescription Drugs*, and is the co-author of the bestselling *The Encyclopedia of Natural Medicine*.